Health in 1980–1990

# 6 | Perspectives in Medicine

General Editor: Leo van der Reis, M.D., San Francisco, Calif.

Philip Selby

B.A., M.B., B.Chir.

# Health in 1980–1990
## A Predictive Study Based on an International Inquiry

Sponsored by
The Henry Dunant Institute of the Red Cross, Geneva,
and
Sandoz Ltd, Basle

S. Karger      1974
Basel · München · Paris · London · New York · Sydney

Perspectives in Medicine

S. Karger AG · Basel · München · Paris · London · New York · Sydney
Arnold-Böcklin-Strasse 25, CH−4011 Basel (Switzerland)

©    Copyright 1974 by S. Karger AG, Verlag für Medizin und Naturwissenschaften, Basel
     Printed in Switzerland by Thür AG Offsetdruck, Pratteln
     ISBN 3−8055−1778−5

# Contents

*To
the memory of
Pierre Boissier*

# Preface

Health is one of man's oldest and most universal preoccupations. Today, demands for better and more extensive health care, encouraged by the rapid progress of medical science and technology and by innovations in health care delivery, are accompanied by a new and widespread curiosity about possible future developments. Moreover, the making of rational and well-founded predictions is of vital interest to health ministries, the medical and allied health professions, economists, sociologists, and diverse other professional groups, as well as to the Red Cross and the pharmaceutical industry.

The Red Cross has, in many countries, its own hospitals, clinics, rehabilitation centres, and numerous other types of care facilities. It collects more than 40 % of the blood donated throughout the world; it operates nursing schools; and it organizes a vast and growing range of training courses on many topics, notably first aid, hygiene, and disease and accident prevention. Certain basic questions must be faced, however, as to the role of the Red Cross over the coming decades; for example, what needs it will have to satisfy, what new areas it should enter, and what it should leave to the State. Its future activities are inseparably linked to the future of health care.

The pharmaceutical industry, too, has a fundamental interest in the future of medicine in the broadest sense of the term, and in planning for the needs of individuals and the community in the years ahead. The position which it occupies in the field of health entails heavy responsibilities towards the public, the health professions, and the State. The formulation of policies in keeping with these responsibilities, rather than dictated by purely commercial considerations, must be based on the forecasting of future needs.

It is therefore not surprising that Sandoz Ltd and the Henry Dunant Institute, the research body of the International Red Cross, joined forces to undertake a predictive study. The fruits of this effort are presented in the pages which follow.

In the Introduction following this Preface, the reader will find a description of the methods used in the study, which involved the collaboration of 63 eminent specialists. We owe the latter our deepest gratitude for their generosity in contributing their valuable time and knowledge, for their patience in answering our questionnaires, and for the endurance displayed by those who participated in the final symposium.

The entire documentation collected during the study, including all the views expressed by the experts consulted, was submitted to Dr Philip Selby, who was not involved in the actual inquiry and who had, at that time, no links with either the Red Cross or the pharmaceutical industry. Dr Selby's task was to carry out, on a wholly independent basis, a final analysis of the material and to present the results of our study in a lucid, readable, and lively manner. We thank him for undertaking and fulfilling that task.

Henry Dunant Institute                                              Sandoz Ltd


*The further investigation of many problems discussed in this book will be among the activities of a newly created institute in Geneva: the Sandoz Institute for Health and Socio-Economic Studies.*

# Introduction

In 1970, the Henry Dunant Institute of the Red Cross, in Geneva, and the pharmaceutical company of Sandoz Ltd, in Basle, embarked on a joint study aiming to predict how health care will be organized in 1980–1990. The study, which was limited to the industrialized countries, was oriented primarily towards the social and economic implications of developments in health care, while not ignoring their purely technological aspects.

The study was based on the so-called Delphi method, which combines certain advantages of a questionnaire survey with other advantages of a round-table conference. The Delphi method, which originated over twenty years ago at the Rand Corporation in the USA, has developed rapidly during the past decade under the stimulus of a world-wide vogue for long-range forecasting as an aid to planning, in particular by large commercial enterprises. The method consists of sending a questionnaire to a number of experts and making a synthesis of their replies to each question. The syntheses are then distributed among the same experts, who have an opportunity of modifying their views in the light of opinions expressed by their fellow experts. A second synthesis is made and the process is repeated. After three or four such exchanges, a final document is prepared expressing all the points on which a consensus may have been reached as well as divergent views. The questionnaire method has the advantages of anonymity and of allowing ample time for reflection, which some individuals prefer. Furthermore, it can sometimes be more successful than a round-table conference in enabling a consensus to be reached on particular problems. At the same time the method, like a conference, allows the interchange of views and ideas.

The greatest value of the Delphi method seems to lie in using intuitive judgement, in other words well-informed guess-work, to produce probability forecasts. The Rand Corporation believes that it marks the beginning of a whole new field of research, which it labels 'opinion technology'. In all areas of futurology, predictions can be proved or disproved by time alone and are at the mercy of the unexpected, for example unforeseen social and political changes or breakthroughs in science and technology. Future innovations in medicine may produce far-reaching changes comparable with those resulting from the introduction of the sulfonamides and antibiotics.

The Red Cross – Sandoz study consisted of a Delphi-type inquiry in two stages, followed one year later by a symposium. The first questionnaire was so designed and worded as to enable the experts to express themselves on those subjects that seemed to them most interesting and on which they felt they could make a useful contribution. For this reason, each expert was given the opportunity of answering as many or as few of the questions as he wished, rather than confining his replies to his own particular specialty. In preparing the first synthesis, an attempt was made to identify the topics that received most attention and those points of view that appeared the most likely to stimulate a further useful exchange of opinion. The synthesis of the replies to each question was divided into three parts: firstly, a brief summary of the general consensus of opinion, where one existed; secondly, a statement of the majority view, not necessarily where more than half of the experts were in agreement but where there seemed to be a strong element of agreement; and thirdly, those minority viewpoints that seemed especially interesting or that tended to conflict with those of the majority. This scheme was not possible for every question, for example those in which no majority viewpoint emerged.

In the second questionnaire the experts were asked to comment on the first synthesis, and in addition to answer a number of new questions arising from the responses to the first questionnaire. Thus while the first questionnaire set the framework for the inquiry, the aims of the second were to try to achieve a consensus of opinion on those points where there was already some agreement, and to probe more deeply into areas that seemed the most interesting or controversial.

Sixty-two experts, from 19 countries of the developed world, participated in these first two stages of the inquiry (see list on p. 83). They represented a wide range of disciplines, including clinical medicine, public health, economics, sociology, medical journalism, and futurology. Unfortunately, there were few participants from Eastern European countries and none from the USSR.

The third stage of the inquiry consisted of a three-day symposium held in Basle, in September 1972. The 16 participants were, with one exception, drawn from among the 62 experts who had taken part in the questionnaire stages of the survey. Their selection was made in such a way as to ensure, as far as possible, a well-balanced interdisciplinary representation. Although a symposium does not form part of the Delphi method, such a gathering was prompted by two considerations. Firstly, the classical type of Delphi study, consisting of three or four exchanges of opinions, is a lengthy procedure which can last for years; and secondly, owing to the vast scope of the subject, it was felt that a live discussion would provide an excellent forum in which to explore certain more interesting points in greater depth. In all stages of the inquiry, the experts were asked to make predictions rather than giving their views on what would be desirable.

The present book, which is an analysis of the preceding study, is based on the experts' replies to the two questionnaires and a verbatim record of the symposium. It follows from the foregoing remarks that such a book cannot aspire to present an overall consensus view, for no such consensus exists; the nature of the subject also precludes the formulation of precise and quantifiable predictions. Moreover, the material obtained in the course of the study touches upon virtually every aspect of health care, without treating any topic in great depth. With these limitations in mind, the positive aims of the book must be emphasized. The author's objective has been to construct a coherent picture of the future of health care which conforms, as far as possible, with the views of most of the experts. He has taken account not only of majority views, but also of those points that seemed to be of greatest importance and interest, even though certain ideas may have come from only one expert.

From this methodology it follows that the views expressed are not necessarily those of the author; neither can he accept responsibility for the accuracy of statistics and other factual material presented. Any criticism must be for his selection and interpretation of the material, and for his attempts to draw meaningful conclusions. Some readers may disagree with these interpretations or conclusions. If the book proves controversial, so much the better. Rather than being the end-point of an inquiry it could, hopefully, become the starting point for further useful discussion.

*Geneva,*                                                                 P.M.S.
*January 1974*

# Health and Disease

# 1 | Major Health Problems

*Three Challenges to Health:*
*Cancer, Cardiovascular Diseases, and Mental Illness*

Man's change from a food-gatherer to a subsistence farmer, and later to a dweller in ever-larger cities, has taken place over a period of some 300 generations. This period is far too brief for genetic change and natural selection to have appreciably altered his racial constitution. Yet the changes are accelerating at breath-taking speed. Only during the last two generations has agriculture, the original basis of civilization, given way to industrialization, while the economically developed part of the world began to enter the post-industrial era less than twenty years ago. The artificial life of modern man, contrasting sharply with the life-style that conditioned his evolution, is fraught with many dangers to his health due to problems of adjusting to the rapidly occurring changes in his physical, social, and emotional environment. Indeed, were it not for man's astonishing adaptability and genetic diversity, one wonders whether he could have survived up to the present time. Yet the dangers are multiplying as it becomes increasingly difficult for his adaptive mechanisms to keep pace.

Man has always depended on his wits to protect himself from external enemies; the history of medicine is a fascinating story of success of this kind in his defence against infection. But he has been conspicuously less successful in his efforts to combat enemies arising within himself due to the impact of his environment and living habits, in the shape of cardiovascular diseases and mental disorders. These two problems, together with malignant diseases, will be the main challenge facing medicine in the developed world for at least the next twenty years.

To meet this challenge the emphasis will shift to prevention. By 1980, public health services will have started carrying out routine prophylactic examinations of the entire population with the aim of detecting disease at a treatable stage. Eventually, complete medical files will be kept on the health of each individual and periodically brought up to date with the aid of computers and automated methods. By 1990, mass screening will extend not only to diseases but to their predisposing factors. Morbidity rates will show an artificial rise due to the early detection of previously unrecognized disease, but hopefully the result will be earlier and more effective treatment, with a lowering of mortality and an increase in life expectancy.

## Cancer

According to the 'iceberg theory', only a small fraction of the total morbidity in a population is clinically recognized. Detection campaigns should therefore lead to an apparent rise in the incidence of malignancies, as well as of other diseases for which screening is carried out. However, the amount of latent disease can only roughly be estimated by viewing the tip of the iceberg. Added uncertainty stems from the difficulty in deciding at what stage early cellular changes can be considered to be actually or potentially malignant. Where is the dividing line, for example, between squamous metaplasia of the cervix and pre-invasive carcinoma? The obscure and insidious origins of cancer will continue to thwart medical science for many years to come.

By 1980, highly sensitive biochemical reactions will permit early detection by revealing changes in the serum, and some ten years later it will be possible to detect malignant changes at the intracellular level. Specific immunological, chromosomal, and enzymatic tests will be developed for diagnosing malignant tumours.

Evidence is mounting that some forms of cancer are caused by viruses. For example, virus particles have been detected in the milk of certain groups of women known to have a high incidence of breast cancer, notably Parsee women in India, and women in the USA who appear to belong to high-risk families. During the 1980's, tumour prophylaxis by vaccines will become a reality; some of these vaccines will also be used in therapy, as will other virostatic agents, such as interferon. While more effective cytostatic agents will be developed, and further innovations made in radiotherapy, these forms of therapy will come to appear relatively crude and will be gradually phased out. A breakthrough can be expected around 1990, with the introduction of antiviral chemotherapy for certain types of cancer.

With a rapid expansion of immunology during the 1980's, biological and chemical agents will be developed to induce immunity against the viruses responsible for certain cancers. Subsequent knowledge of the mechanisms by which some forms of cancer develop will lead to methods of immunological surveillance for use in early detection and for the follow-up of known cases. Certain anti-tumour sera may be shown to be effective in immunotherapy by about 1990, while immunotherapy and chemotherapy will be developed against specific nucleic acids. Tumour surgery will continue to have a place, but a more limited one, often in conjunction with immunotherapy.

Lung cancer well illustrates the iceberg theory, the diagnosis in some 90 % of cases being made too late for any treatment to be of avail. At the same time, it shows up some of the current difficulties involved in carrying out preventive measures. Screening programmes using present methods – bronchoscopy, radiography, tomography, and cytology – would be time-consuming and expensive; indeed, the question of cost-benefit ratio constitutes one of the limitations confronting preventive medicine. The advent of specific serological tests for the early detection of cancers will radically transform the potential of mass screening programmes, especially if, as is highly likely, these tests can be performed by automated methods. The prevention of lung cancer also indicates a second problem, requiring a different solution, namely, that even when a specific environmental factor is known to contribute to a disease, attempts to remove the offending cause are thwarted by man's tenacious adherence to established customs and attitudes. Anti-smoking campaigns have had remarkably little impact on smoking habits. Moreover, the attitude of smokers is often tinged with an extraordinary degree of fatalism; one has to die of something, so why give up a pleasurable habit? With recently increased awareness of the dangers, the first halting steps in prevention have been taken. An energetic drive can be foreseen over the coming years in the form of more intensive anti-smoking campaigns, even extending to the total prohibition of the sale of cigarettes in some countries.

For some unknown reason, cancer of the stomach is becoming slightly less common in Europe and the USA, while its prevalence continues to rise in Japan. Although attempts have been made to incriminate dietary practices, in particular the consumption of salty and smoked foods, the disease is, curiously enough, just as frequent among second-generation Japanese living in the USA, who have completely adopted the Western diet. Rigorous attempts are being made in Japan to detect this killing disease early enough to give some hope of treatment. Among these is endoscopy, using highly sophisticated techniques which yield remarkably clear photographs of early lesions long before symptoms develop or radiology would show any abnormality. Yet the systematic and regular screening of entire populations by this method is laborious, not to say unpleasant. Here again, serological tests will revolutionize early detection campaigns.

Breast cancer is another disease where future hopes lie less in cure than in prevention. Despite a multilateral attack via surgery, chemotherapy, and hormone therapy, effective treatment for most cases has not yet been found. Neither does earlier detection hold great promise; according to one estimate, 98 % of cases are already incurable even when the lesion is detected at a diameter of about 1 cm. Compounding the problem is the refusal of many women, based on fear, to examine their own breasts, even though this is easy to do and the prognosis would perhaps be improved by early detection. However, the long-term effects of early detection campaigns, such as those carried out in New York, remain to be seen. Because of the ever-present consideration of cost-versus-benefits, attention may well be focused on high-risk groups: women with a family history of breast cancer; women who started menstruating early and produced a child relatively late in life; and women who are childless or have never breast-fed. In women with a racial or familial predisposition, prevention may be more effective than early detection, firstly by counselling against breast-feeding, and secondly, through vaccination once this becomes available.

As a result of developments in prevention, early detection, and treatment such as those outlined above, it is likely that, although malignant disease will still be a major problem in twenty years' time, some 70 % of cancers will at least be controllable by then.

Cardiovascular Diseases

Tomorrow's solutions to cardiovascular diseases will be extensions of today's partial answers. Since many predisposing factors are known, the way is already open to prevention, particularly through early detection programmes and the wider application of health education. Moreover, the lines of future research, and of developments in drug therapy and surgical techniques, seem clearly drawn for at least the next twenty years.

The dangers of obesity and a sedentary life will, from the changing nature of man's environment, tend to increase over this period. The ratio of population to food supply will not have begun to act as a curb on the gluttony of man in the developed world, neither will fuel shortages have reached the point where he is obliged to resume the use of his legs as a means of transport. Prevention, therefore, will require an awareness of the problems, followed by a conscious choice on the part of the individual. To promote awareness, health education programmes in schools, factories, and other places of work, as well as via the mass media, will emphasize healthy nutrition and the active use of leisure time, including sport, not as an occasional means of escape but as an integral part of everyday life. The drive to reduce cigarette smoking will further help to prevent cardiovascular disease.

Mass early detection campaigns will identify those individuals at high risk, on whom preventive measures can be focused. Thus, screening will be carried out for predisposing genetic and environmental factors; methods will be developed for the early detection of atherosclerosis; the blood pressure of the entire population will be checked routinely; and by 1980, children and young adults will routinely be screened for abnormal levels of blood lipids. During the 1980's atheroma will become a preventable condition, and it will also be possible to arrest its progress; methods will include nutritional control, the correction of high blood lipid levels and glycoprotein disturbances, and specific drugs. A drug for lowering the blood cholesterol level will be developed by about 1975.

New types of therapy will include the treatment of obesity by effective agents that burn off excess calories without causing adverse reactions; a long-acting drug for the control of angina pectoris which modifies the needs of the myocardium; and drugs for controlling cardiac action in order to combat the effects of stress when necessary, to prevent emotional 'overloading'. Not before 1990 will the precise cause or causes of essential hypertension be identified, permitting safe and effective preventive or therapeutic control.

The next twenty years will see the successful development of surgical techniques that are today at an early and experimental stage. Surgery of the coronary arteries, for example, will be widely practised by the late 1970's. It will be some ten years later, however, before the same will be true of artificial heart implants and heart transplants from animal donors. But in all probability the dream of rejuvenating atherosclerotic arteries will never be realized.

Mental Illness

Statistics for the past few years show a remarkable rise in the prevalence of mental illness. But are they a valid indication of future trends? Many such diseases are increasing as a result of social changes, the future evolution of which is open to speculation; as these changes appear to be taking place with increasing rapidity, society may be heading for a crisis situation, or at least for widespread social upheavals. Moreover, are the figures to be believed? While statistics in general may be misleading, those relating to mental illness can be especially unreliable, since no objective biological or other test is available for diagnosing these conditions; diagnosis is based on a subjective clinical impression together with society's failure to tolerate certain types of behaviour. Some such statistics are quite impressive: 20 % of students at English universities suffer from some mental disorder at some stage during the course of their studies; only 35 % of a French rural population that was studied were free of any psychiatric disorder, while a quarter of the subjects had a frankly diminished mental capacity; in a Canadian study of 400,000 subjects from all socio-economic classes, only 20 % showed no mental disturbance; and the largest study so far carried out in New York, on 200,000 subjects, revealed some type of neurosis in 43 % of individuals from the wealthy classes, compared with 25 % among the poorer classes, with a prevalence of psychoses of 4 % and 13 %, respectively. Statistics such as these may lead one to the broad conclusion that half the population of the Western world is mentally ill, and that the neuroses are more prevalent among the upper classes while the psychoses are commoner among the lower classes.

Statistics from the French national health insurance scheme approach the type of objectivity we are looking for. Declarations of incapacity for work, carrying the right to sickness benefits, are based not only on the diagnosis made by the patient's own doctor, but on a careful scrutiny of each case by physicians employed on behalf of the insurance scheme. They can thus reasonably be equated with the individual's incapacity to play a productive role in society. In the 20-year period from 1950 to 1970, these statistics for France as a whole show a four-fold increase in the number of annual declarations of incapacity for work due to mental illness, an increase which is comparable to that in England and certain other industrialized countries. These same statistics also show that, at the end of this period, some 25 % of all cases of incapacity for work in the Paris region, and some 22 % in the country as a whole, were due to mental illness. By contrast, the proportion of cases due to tuberculosis fell from 27 % to 4 % in France during the 20-year period, while that due to cancer and cardiovascular diseases showed no significant change.

However imprecise our means of quantifying the changing pattern of mental illness, the problem is quite evidently growing at an alarming rate. Let us now take a separate look at two categories of mental illness, the psychoses and the neuroses.

*Psychoses*

Tomorrow's answers to dealing with the psychoses appear to lie mainly in finding biochemical solutions to their causes, diagnosis, and treatment. During the 1980's, progress will be made in the early detection of schizophrenia and certain other psychoses, and in their prevention in persons found to be at risk. A major advance will be the introduction of chemotherapy, around the year 1990, following the discovery of the bio-chemical causes of certain psychoses, including schizophrenia. Quite possibly, a number of psychoses will be found to be due to enzymic distur-bances; a parallel may be drawn between the present state of knowledge about them and what was understood about diabetes in the pre-insulin era. Their treatment may evolve along similar lines, combined with social intervention where necessary. Probably not before the turn of the cen-tury, if ever, will specific chemical diagnostic tests and individual drugs be available for each biochemical lesion causing mental illness.

*Neuroses*

If the causes for psychiatric consultations are analysed, it becomes evident that the rapid and continuing rise in the prevalence of mental disorders is due entirely to an increase in neuroses. The rising curve, which is similar in all industrialized countries, is roughly keeping pace with the growth of urbanization. It stems from a number of causes. Overcrowding in huge cities leads to ever-greater stress and 'psychological pollution', with difficulties or even total failure of adaptation. Rural populations migrating into urban areas are particularly ill-equipped to cope with the exigencies of the urban way of life, and to adapt to completely different working and living conditions. When the individual's compensatory mech-anisms fail, stress disorders ensue. It has sometimes been claimed, though not proved, that certain behavioural problems, such as drug abuse, aggres-sions, attempted suicide, and sexual deviations, may result from such failure. Increasingly, recourse is made to psychotropic drugs such as stimu-lants, tranquillizers, and anti-depressants; these will be discussed in more detail in a later chapter. In addition, the citizen is subjected to ever-greater pressures due to the attitudes of a society that places emphasis on achieve-ment and self-fulfilment, in a context of competitiveness among solitary individuals who are isolated from one another in the crowd. The sharp drop in neuroses during the Second World War, and their subsequent rise in peace-time, is a striking illustration of this process.

The psychological influence of changes in working conditions was well shown by certain consequences that followed modernization of the

French national railways. In the days of steam engines, the mechanics, whose task was physically exhausting, hardly ever showed signs of psychological decompensation. Following the change-over to electric locomotives, however, a remarkable number of neuroses and psychosomatic disorders were observed. A series of enquiries made among these workers showed that they complained, firstly, of no longer having to make the physical effort that formerly had provided a bond between them and their machines. Secondly, they found it intolerable to be subjected to what they called the judgement of a machine; that is to say, their working performance was reflected in the responses of an inanimate mechanism rather than by the reactions of their fellow mechanics. With the rapid changes of modern industrial society, similar innovations are revolutionizing the working lives of millions of citizens.

Adding further to the problem of mental disorders is the aging population of the industrialized countries, due mainly to improved health care and a falling birth rate. Over the past 100 years, the proportion of the population over the age of 60 years has tripled in all European countries, while the proportion over the age of 80 years has shown a five-fold increase. Within one more generation, 25 % of the populations of many countries, for example Sweden and the USA, may be over the age of 60 years. Psychological problems arise in the elderly from the sudden cessation of work, and hence education for an active retirement will be an important aspect of preventive medicine. Further, the physical and social structure of large cities, and the breakdown of traditional family ties, are causing old people to become increasingly isolated and lonely, with ensuing problems such as anxiety and depression.

Finally, the threshold of tolerance in modern society has been lowered, so that minor forms of psychological deviation are now considered to need medical treatment. Medicine is expected to provide solutions to behavioural problems and difficulties of adaptation, no less than to varicose veins or diabetes.

Short of a radical and purposeful re-structuring of society, which seems highly improbable at least in this century, man will show increasing failure to adapt to his environment. This process of decompensation is at the root of the prodigious rise in neurotic illness. It is manifest, firstly, by difficulties in interpersonal relations, or even their breakdown, the signs of which are already clear in certain large cities in the USA; and secondly, by failure to adapt to society, with concomitant behavioural problems such as drug abuse and attempted suicide. Here, perhaps, a note of caution is needed; adaptation to a particular society, or failure to adapt, is sometimes a matter of cultural definition. From time to time men arise with revolutionary ideas in the field of politics, philosophy, or science, who challenge the concepts and values of the society in which they live. Such diversity, far from being pathological, is in fact one of society's most vital assets, which may help it to avoid or weather its approaching crises just as genetic diversity has enabled the human species to adapt and survive up to the present time. In this context, many people view with misgivings the repression of those holding dissident opinions.

How will the medical profession, and psychiatrists in particular, cope with the growing problem? In terms of sheer numbers of neurotic or maladapted people, it is clear that soon there will not be enough psychiatrists to deal with these cases along traditional lines. The emphasis will shift from the care of individual patients to the mental health of populations, to group therapy and health education of communities. To this end, the training of psychiatrists and other mental health workers will undergo fundamental changes, with the introduction of new approaches based on sociological and political concepts. Since many reactional neuroses are due to family or working conditions, the general practitioner and the industrial physician will be given a more thorough training in the origins and, particularly, the prevention of these conditions. Because of the inadequacy of medical resources in the face of growing needs, many problems, especially those connected with behavioural disturbances, will have to be solved by self-help and assistance within the family group, for example by transactional analysis. This is not to suggest that psychoanalysis will disappear; on the contrary, its use is expanding enormously in the USA, and it may well do so in other countries among those sectors of the population who can afford it. Nevertheless, the next twenty years may well be a period of undreamed-of development in family medicine and the activation of people in the solution of their own problems.

Emotional disorders of childhood deserve special mention, recent studies indicating that some 7 % of all children, and 10 % of adolescents, are in need of assistance for severe emotional distress. While prospective studies are required to define the positive and negative effects of environmental factors in emotional development, many of these disorders clearly result from disturbances of the parent-child relationship. Doctors, mental health workers, and educational psychologists will in future be trained to diagnose and deal with this type of problem. Likewise, all those coming into contact with young children, including infant welfare workers, kindergarten supervisors, and schoolteachers, will be alerted to detecting disturbances in parent-child interaction at the earliest possible moment. In an attempt to find a more radical solution, a great deal of research will be devoted to the development of healthy child-rearing practices, followed by efforts to instruct and motivate parents in the adoption of these practices.

## Some Other Health Problems

### The Aging Process

Since earliest times man has dreamed of immortality. While he is unlikely ever to achieve this ambition, he has succeeded in prolonging his life expectancy through advances in medical care and improved living conditions. This success, together with falling birth rates, is responsible for the continued aging of populations in the developed world, as a result of which the health problems of old age are assuming ever-greater importance. During the coming years, attempts will be made to prevent, slow down, or even reverse those degenerative changes that are due to the aging process, in order to achieve not merely a longer old age but a more healthy one.

During the next ten years, progress will be made in preventing or delaying the onset of cerebral atrophy and senile dementia, and of senile osteoporosis and anaemias. A start will be made in developing methods, beginning at birth, for delaying the aging process. A radical approach to prevention will have to wait until the basic causes of the aging process have been further elucidated and cannot be foreseen within the next twenty years. Education in physical and mental hygiene, based on what is known of the normal aging process, will be widely disseminated; it will encourage healthy nutrition, exercise, and certain forms of drug therapy for high-risk cases, and will teach people how to prepare themselves for old age. Treatment will develop on many fronts, involving all the disciplines of medicine; endocrine therapy, for example, will be tried during the 1980's. For those who are afflicted by the scourge of senile decay, and whose health needs are the greatest, supportive health care will include social measures such as adequate housing, social security, and free health insurance.

### Genetically Determined Diseases

Progress in genetic engineering will be made over the next few decades, but its use in the treatment and antenatal prevention of inherited

# 2 | Prevention

Within the next twenty years factory and office workers will take regular breaks for calisthenics, while physical culture and sport will be encouraged among all age groups and all sectors of the community. As leisure time expands, owing to shorter working hours and earlier retirement, greater efforts will be made to ensure its active use in such a way as to promote health and prevent disease. Such developments will form one aspect of the growing emphasis on prevention in health care. New and far-reaching preventive health policies, to be conceived during the coming decade, will also include the promotion of health education, occupational health, and immunization and early detection programmes. They will be based on further research in epidemiology, for example concerning the relationship between environmental factors and cardiovascular diseases, the neuroses, the pneumoconioses, and some endocrine disorders.

Health education in schools and via the mass media will emphasize the harmful effects of drug abuse, alcohol, tobacco, and unhealthy nutritional practices, as well as advising on how to utilize the health services most effectively. Propaganda campaigns aimed at preserving the quality of the environment will be stepped up, using methods taken from the world of commercial advertising and publicity. A long and concerted effort will be needed, however, to produce a responsible attitude towards environmental protection throughout the entire population.

Since education, in a democratic society, is based on persuasion rather than coercion, it will produce results slowly. Rapid advances, on the other hand, will be seen in occupational health, largely because economic considerations, such as greater efficiency and reduced costs of absenteeism, will motivate employers to participate actively in preventive measures and the improvement of working conditions. Certain occupational diseases, such as the pneumoconioses and some cancers, will be largely eliminated, while industrial accidents will be drastically reduced.

diseases will still be a dream by 1990. The enormous risks involved
research may lead to severe mishaps from early attempts to use it, c
parable in magnitude with the one due to thalidomide. Strict control
therefore be exercised over such work, by public authorities and the m
cal profession. Chemical, physical, and viral methods will all be tried.

On the other hand, the rapid development of research into gen
mechanisms will soon make it possible to predict inherited diseases, le
ing to a great upsurge in genetic counselling. The concept of a 'gen
identity card' and the question of sterilizing carriers of certain harn
genes will provoke serious discussion; a gradual ethical evolution is pi
able towards the acceptance of eugenics in preventing some types of dise

Mongolism and certain other genetic disorders will be detected
*utero* by the examination of cells aspirated by amniocentesis, mak
prevention possible by therapeutic abortion.

### Viral Diseases

A massive onslaught against the viral diseases will be launched d
the next twenty years. By 1980, besides a wide variety of more effec
vaccines, there will be a universal virus vaccine and a vaccine against sei
hepatitis which, given routinely, will reduce this disease to the same
tent that has occurred with poliomyelitis. By that date, too, there may
compulsory vaccination against influenza, measles, and rubella in
before the age of puberty, leading to the eradication of these disease
some countries. The range of compulsory vaccinations will later be
tended to all communicable viral diseases. By 1990, forms of interven
will include chemotherapy, chemoprophylaxis, and methods of stimu
ing interferon production by the body.

### Venereal Diseases

Attempts to curb the rapid increase in venereal diseases will be n
through health education and sex education, particularly in school
seems highly unlikely that this will lead to an era of sexual austerity ir
Western world, as occurred in China as a result of the social transfo
tions after 1948. Furthermore, the chances of its reducing sexual pe
siveness will be effectively scotched, during the 1980's, by the intro
tion of vaccines, which may quite well have the contrary effect. In tw
years' time there may well be a permissive society that is relatively
from venereal diseases.

The attack on communicable diseases during the next twenty years will be based on mass immunization against an increasing number of viral diseases, notably influenza, measles, rubella, and hepatitis, while vaccines will also be developed against the venereal diseases and certain cancers. Substances will be discovered that increase the body's non-specific resistance to various types of potentially harmful factor, from bacteria and viruses to toxins and noise.

Preventive medicine will take a great leap forward with the widespread adoption of early detection programmes. In the face of ever-increasing demands for health care, multiphasic screening will prove a highly efficient method for separating out malingerers and hypochondriacs from true pathological cases and from subclinical cases who are at risk of acquiring a disease. The detection of high-risk cases will enable preventive measures to be applied, while the early detection of diseases will lead to earlier and more effective treatment; hence the links between preventive and curative medicine will become ever closer. Early detection will comprise a continuum of three methods, each having slightly different objectives: the health check-up, multiphasic screening, and the more detailed health evaluation and follow-up of high-risk cases.

The health check-up consists of a number of simple tests. The means may be developed whereby these can be carried out by the subject himself in his own home. If such means are not available, the tests will be carried out by the general practitioner or allied health personnel, often in the district preventive medicine centre. They will screen for easily detected conditions such as obesity, diabetes, hypertension, and albuminuria. By the end of this decade, regular check-ups will be encouraged for the whole population at intervals of a year, six months, or even less. In some cases they will be obligatory, for example as a condition for employment. Clearly, they will involve a considerable demand on health manpower.

Multiphasic screening, already in use, will expand widely and rapidly over the coming years. Most probably it will be applied first to certain categories of the population, for example preschool children or persons over the age of 55 years, before being extended to the entire population. While its primary aims will be the early detection of diseases and the identification of high-risk cases, it will also provide a vast amount of statistics for use in epidemiological research. Data will be obtained by a variety of methods. Questionnaires will provide information on predisposing factors such as smoking, diet, and family history. Automated, multi-channel analysers will perform differential blood cell counts, as well as tests based on biochemical, immunological, and enzymic reactions; by the late 1980's, such methods will help in the detection of certain mental disorders. Biophysical methods will include the use of radioisotopes, ultrasonics, and thermography, while X-rays and cytology smears will be read by computers. Tests of hepatic, renal, cardiovascular, pulmonary, and cerebral functions will include dynamic testing under some kind of load; for example, the way certain chemical substances are detoxified and eliminated from the body may indicate a tendency to develop hypertension. Screening may well extend to certain psychological tests too, for example to detect learning difficulties in schoolchildren.

The efficiency and workability of multiphasic screening will stem from the use of auto-analysers, enabling accurately standardized tests to be carried out rapidly and cheaply on an enormous number of subjects, together with the use of computers in the interpretation of results. Through the collection and correlation of a wide variety of data, a health profile will be drawn for each individual on which danger signs can be noted. On the basis of deviations from population norms, and changes observed in successive examinations, computers will provide a differential diagnosis and an estimate of the size of risk involved. While serving as a valuable tool, such methods will not preclude the need for clinical interpretation of the results, which according to traditional belief is more an art than a science. Machines cannot provide an automatic diagnosis, but merely the automatic processing of data to facilitate the making of a diagnosis. Computer technology cannot, therefore, be regarded as a panacea. The ways in which it can best be applied to health care need to be clearly defined through further studies.

Once a high-risk case is identified, a precise health evaluation of the individual will be made by clinical examination and a battery of specific tests. These will be interpreted by the clinician in personal contact with the patient, who will also decide what preventive or therapeutic measures are needed. Preventive measures will consist of attempts to remove known contributory factors, for example through a change of occupation, with therapy in some cases to prevent the onset of the threatening disease or to slow its progress. Follow-up will require repeat health evaluations at regular intervals. Clearly, for such a system to work properly, both doctors and patients must be convinced of the importance of follow-up procedures even in the absence of overt disease or disability.

This new type of medicine should produce such striking early results as to win the enthusiastic support of clinicians, public health workers, epidemiologists, and the population as a whole. Any initial resistance on the part of the public to participation will not only disappear, but will give way to popular demand for the fullest possible development of screening and follow-up programmes. Added to the benefits deriving from more effective disease prevention, these programmes will also provide a tremendous saving of the doctor's time. Within the next ten years their impact will be felt throughout the entire organization and practice of medicine.

Because of their high costs and their application to large numbers of people, and eventually the entire population, automated and computerized methods for disease detection and diagnosis will be organized and financed almost entirely within the public health sector. On a more limited scale, large industries may provide internal automated health services for their employees, while some university departments, backed by private finance, may offer early diagnostic testing for individuals who are willing to pay the price. In countries where attempts are already being made by private organizations to supply computer services in the diagnostic and therapeutic areas, they are meeting a cautious response from governments and the medical profession. Collaboration may develop between the public and private sectors. In the USA and other non-socialist countries, studies, experiments, and early implementation could be carried out in the private sector with heavy government subsidies, followed by progressive integration into the health services in accordance with governmental planning and performance criteria. Services will most likely remain under the control of whoever bears the cost of health care. In the USA, this could be a universal health insurance programme with federal financing and guidelines, along the lines of the Medicare programme. Automation and computer technology are likely to develop in a more or less disorganized way over the next decade or two. Not until around 1990 will joint efforts by the State and private research centres bring about their effective co-ordination within the health services.

Since the rationale for screening programmes is based on the so-called 'iceberg theory', it is worth examining the submerged part of the iceberg more closely. In so far as we relate this to early detection in the true sense, it consists of latent, subclinical disease that has hitherto passed unrecognized both by the affected individuals and by those responsible for their health care. From a practical point of view, it also includes clinical conditions that have remained untreated, either because of some people's reluctance to seek medical advice until driven to do so by severe discomfort or incapacity, or as a result of inadequate access to medical care in some low-income areas. From the standpoint of community health, undetected or untreated disease is of greatest importance when it is both communicable and treatable, for example pulmonary tuberculosis. As far as the individual is concerned, the greatest tragedy occurs when delay in treatment proves lethal, as with certain forms of cancer, or produces some permanent disability that might have been avoided, for example glaucoma or diabetes.

Just how big is the submerged part of the iceberg? As regards untreated clinical disease, a number of surveys have shown the prevalence to vary greatly from one place to another, from one type of disease to another, and between socio-economic, cultural, and educational groups. The amount of subclinical disease, on the other hand, will only gradually be revealed over the coming years through mass screening programmes. While a diagnosis of subclinical abnormality will be based, not on an isolated test, but on the analysis of one or several successive health profiles, the number of cases detected will be influenced by the values that are selected as borderline between normal and abnormal. Does one choose, for example, a diastolic blood pressure of 90, 95, or 100 mm Hg? Or a serum cholesterol level of 220, 260, or 300 mg %? Nevertheless, the fact that it is often some complication which leads to the diagnosis of chronic diseases, such as hepatic failure, cancer, atherosclerosis, gout, and diabetes, suggests that the amount of subclinical disease may turn out to be very large.

The bigger the hidden part of the iceberg, the greater is the potential public health value of mass screening programmes. Like all health programmes, however, they will have to compete for financing with other projects, owing to the limited size of the health budget. Health planners will soon face the difficult task of assessing the cost of such programmes and the economic returns to be expected. While the cost of setting up mass screening programmes can be calculated fairly accurately, in terms of equipment, facilities, and personnel, their economic consequences are shrouded in uncertainty, firstly, because we do not yet know how much iceberg lies below the surface, and secondly, because the economic effects of early treatment cannot be foreseen with any accuracy.

Increased expenditure will be needed to treat clinical disease that is detected and to follow up high-risk cases, while loss of working time for investigations and treatment represents a burden on the national economy. Earlier treatment will sometimes cost less than the treatment of advanced disease, and cut down the total cost of treatment and hospitalization through reducing the duration of illness, its severity, and the number of relapses. In other cases, treatment costs will be expensive even when a disease is detected earlier, for example early detection of breast or uterine cancer leading to surgical intervention. It seems most probable that mass screening programmes will lead to an enormous rise in expenditure in their early stages, whereas economies will follow once the reservoir of untreated and latent disease has been brought under control. This reservoir may prove so large, however, that only a fraction can be followed up adequately with the resources that are available, and consequently it will be a long time before a saving on health expenditure is observed. To the extent that the submerged part of the iceberg is adequately dealt with, the ensuing reduction of sickness and invalidity, and prolongation of working lives, will lead to greater productivity and will thereby represent an economic gain to society as a whole.

# 3 | Treatment

As advances in prevention and treatment bring about changes in the pattern of diseases, as the scourges of today give way to the health threats of tomorrow, so will various types of therapy become unnecessary or be rendered obsolete by newer and better techniques. In this way conventional radiotherapy, for example, will decline over the coming years, and by 1990 will persist only in a limited form employing more refined techniques and new isotopes with more specific and precise effects. In contrast, rapid and spectacular progress will continue to be made in techniques for replacing parts of the body by transplants or artificial devices; while genetic engineering will begin a slow and gradual climb to prominence, one that will continue until well past the turn of the century, and which may or may not achieve eventual success. Efforts will continue to develop immunological and chemotherapeutic methods for the control of malignant disease; in cardiovascular diseases, the most remarkable developments will be in heart and vascular surgery; the tremendous increase in neuroses will stimulate the search for new psychotropic drugs, as well as for ways of correcting psycho-social factors in the environment; while traumatic surgery will develop rapidly under the pressure of a continued increase in the number of road accident victims.

The per capita consumption of pharmaceutical products is likely to double over the next twenty years, largely as a result of more extensive self-medication and the growing use of psychotropic agents. In addition, certain medicaments, while not necessarily effecting a cure, do help to prolong life and thereby to perpetuate consumption; this is true especially with the chronic degenerative diseases of old age. Expenditure on medication is rising as a result of this increasing consumption as well as the higher cost of new drugs. The variety of drugs available is growing rapidly, many new synthetic products being developed that are highly effective and specific, for example new psychotropic agents. The increasing attention being paid to drug action at the cellular level will lead to new delivery systems that allow prolonged therapeutic activity on specific organs or tissues. It will thus be unnecessary to saturate the whole body with a drug when the target area is, for example, the kidney, eye, heart, or basal ganglia. This innovation will lead to greater reliability with fewer systemic and toxic side-effects.

Research in immunology will lead to immunotherapy for the control of some cancers, as well as for the treatment of autoimmune diseases. Great advances will also be made in antiviral chemotherapy and hormone therapy. Spurred on by the rapidly growing problem of mental illness, intensive research in neuro-endocrinology and psycho-pharmacology will lead to the development of agents that are effective in influencing mood, memory, learning ability, and emotional disorders. All types of neuroses will become treatable and perhaps curable, while some of the psychoses will be amenable, if not to cure, at least to improvement and stabilization by drug therapy.

As a result of progress in preventive medicine and therapeutics, certain types of surgery will become far less common or will disappear. The most remarkable effect of this type will be on the surgery of malignant tumours, which may have become almost obsolete by 1990. Surgical removal of vesical and renal calculi will also become unnecessary, once ways are found of dissolving them or preventing their occurrence in high-risk cases that are detected through mass screening programmes. On the other hand, some types of surgery will make spectacular progress, and their technology will evolve rapidly. In traumatic surgery, new adhesive procedures will be developed for speeding the repair of fractures, while around 1990 it will be possible to replace damaged nerves and nerve channels in the spinal cord. Attempts to prevent or slow down the degenerative diseases will be complemented by reparative surgery, notably the replacement or repair of arteriosclerotic vessels, for example the coronary arteries, the more extensive replacement of arthritic joints by prostheses, and the use of tissue transplants. The surgical correction of congenital anomalies will continue to play an important role, helped greatly by new techniques employing miniaturized equipment and the extended use of lasers for delicate repair work. The greatest changes will be seen, however, in the replacement or compensation of defective or useless organs.

The problem of graft rejection will not be completely overcome within the next twenty years, and indeed may never be solved. What progress is made will nevertheless encourage the widespread use of heart, lung, kidney, and liver transplants, in addition to new types of graft such as teeth and blood vessels. By 1990, extensive banks will be kept of human and animal organs and tissues. In parallel with these developments, surgery will focus increasingly on the replacement of body parts using artificial internal organs and prostheses for limbs, joints, and blood vessels. A portable artificial kidney can be expected by the late 1970's, while some ten years later artificial hearts will largely have replaced human or animal transplants. In addition to the replacement of failing organs, compensatory devices will be used, such as heart pumps and pacemakers. By about 1990, it should be technically possible to replace most parts of the body, except the brain and spinal cord, by natural transplants or prostheses, and stocks containing a wide range of artificial organs will be available by the year 2,000. A new concept will be developed, that of the 'cyborg', or cybernetic organism, an individual who can live only in association with some artificial device such as a pacemaker, or an artificial heart or kidney; this will entail new notions of medical care, including attention to the psychological needs of such persons.

The changes described will be accompanied by the development of more refined operation techniques. The wide use of endoscopy will enable smaller incisions to be made, while improved methods will be developed for closing wounds. Greater use will be made of ultrasonics, for example in the localization of stones, tumours, and the placental site, and of bloodless techniques such as cryosurgery in treating Parkinson's disease and certain tumours, such as deep brain tumours and tumours of the prostate and bone.

Finally, a note of caution must be sounded in predicting technological solutions to disease problems. Some, especially the use of organ transplants and implants, are expensive, and must be viewed against a background of conflicting demands upon the health budget. The restraining factor in their development and use may well be, not a lack of ingenuity or scientific expertise, but the limitation of available resources.

# 4 | Rehabilitation

The concept of rehabilitation, up to the present, has been largely restricted to the long, often incomplete process of adjusting handicapped persons to their disability. In the future, however, rehabilitation will be accepted as the essential end-stage of treatment, and as such will play a vital part in the management of all conditions, from the simplest, such as a broken arm or leg, to the most disabling. By the end of the present decade it will form an integral part of the medical care of all patients, including the physically and mentally handicapped and those who have been treated for organic disease or behavioural disorders, such as drug abuse, alcoholism, or delinquency. In keeping with the concept of total medical care, the aims of rehabilitation will extend beyond ensuring the individual's capacity to work and to be independent in his daily life, to achieving fitness for leisure activities and the ability to enjoy life. Thus the next twenty years will see a great expansion of rehabilitation services.

While the number of handicapped persons will continue to rise during the 1980's, this increase will be slowed down by the prevention or treatment of many crippling conditions, such as hereditary, infective, and degenerative diseases of the nervous system, and by measures to prevent industrial and road traffic accidents.

Rehabilitation after treatment for drug abuse and alcoholism merits special consideration, firstly, because the sector of the population that is involved is believed by some to be oriented towards self-destruction and may, therefore, have a high risk of relapse; and secondly, because of the possible causal relationship to social changes. Growing urbanization, leading to psychological and emotional stress, and the expansion of leisure time that is not used purposefully, have been blamed for these and other types of behavioural disorders. If this supposition is true, they will pose a rapidly growing problem, comparable with that presented by the neuroses and emotional disorders. Social measures for rehabilitation will be boosted by the growing emphasis on community care, aided, in the case of behavioural disorders, by further knowledge about their etiology.

As awareness of its importance grows, rehabilitation will come to be accepted as a community responsibility, in particular with regard to the needs of the handicapped. The evolution of social attitudes, and growing governmental concern, will be reflected in new legislation, the expansion of existing services and the development of new ones, and new forms of specialized training for workers in this field. Various programmes will be developed and implemented, producing gradual modifications in the existing health services rather than radical changes. Being one of many aspects of health care, rehabilitation will be carried out within the framework of existing health services in hospitals and health centres. In large hospitals, where medico-surgical departments of cardiology, nephrology, etc., will almost entirely replace today's polyvalent medical and surgical services, it will be provided as the last item of treatment, in a special unit attached to each of these departments.

In addition, rehabilitation and re-adjustment centres will be set up, employing specially trained personnel, for certain categories of patients, such as those who have been treated for myocardial infarction, drug dependence, or alcoholism or who suffer from a motor disability or severe mental handicap. Some 'health cure' resorts will be turned into such centres. An invaluable part of rehabilitation of the handicapped will be provided by sheltered workshops for both children and adults, while a number of permanent homes and villages will be established for handicapped persons of all ages. How soon such facilities appear in any country will depend largely upon the level of economic and social development. While most rehabilitation centres will form part of the government health services, many will be jointly supported by governmental and private bodies. In an attempt to provide the enormous manpower resources that will be required, government-financed training programmes will be expanded. Social workers, for example, will receive higher academic training oriented towards the problems of rehabilitation. The need for intensified rehabilitation services for drug dependence and alcoholism will, indeed, be one of the greatest challenges to social welfare work associated with the rapid growth of urbanization, demanding an expansion of both social case work and group therapy. It is by no means certain that adequate services will be provided, in most countries, during the next twenty years.

Doctors will be increasingly concerned with rehabilitation of the handicapped, especially in fields where the number of such cases is greatest, such as cardiology, crippling conditions of childhood, and certain neurological disorders. Most of the work, however, will be carried out by rehabilitation specialists, large numbers of whom will be needed within the framework of the health services and who will constitute a new and important category of health personnel. Some of these new health professionals will specialize in the rehabilitation of certain types of patients, others in the use of procedures that are applied to different categories, for example special teaching methods. Inevitably, there will never be enough qualified personnel; consequently, they will be helped out by a growing body of volunteers, a trend that is already evident in England and the USA. Just how these volunteers will be deployed must depend on how the rehabilitation services are organized and where the greatest needs exist; they could be used, for example, to help individual handicapped persons in crisis situations. Continuing shortage of personnel, facilities, and equipment for rehabilitation services, together with growing demands, may lead some governments to pay relatives to care for the handicapped at home, helped by visiting health counsellors.

While expenditure on rehabilitation, which depends on national health policies, will vary from one country to another, there will be an overall trend towards a greater portion of the health budget being devoted to this purpose. This trend will arise both from increasing awareness of needs and from economic considerations. The economic benefits are potentially high, in enabling the handicapped to be usefully employed. It may be illusory, however, to expect that countries which suffer from severe under-employment, or crises of unemployment, will be greatly motivated to rehabilitate working people, desirable though this may be from a humanitarian point of view; to this extent, the development of an ethic of rehabilitation may well depend on economic and social factors. Economic benefits, in the form of a direct saving on the costs of health care, will also be derived from thorough and efficient rehabilitation programmes, through reducing the severity of disability and preventing the exacerbation or recurrence of disease. Such programmes may thus prove a good investment when subjected to cost-benefit analysis. In all countries, rehabilitation will need to compete with other demands on the health budget, so that the whole process and its benefits must be subjected to a continuing and critical evaluation.

One effect of the high cost of rehabilitation services will be to encourage the early detection of those conditions for which rehabilitation needs are the greatest, and the identification of high-risk individuals, with the aim of introducing prophylactic measures. Systematic infant and child screening programmes will be set up for the early detection of physical and mental conditions that can cause disability. Attempts will also be made, using biochemical and psychological tests, to identify at an early age individuals with a predisposition to the development of mental illness, alcoholism, or drug dependence. Prospective studies will help in picking out those who are at increased risk as a result of genetic or environmental factors, or because of maladaptation to their environment for whatever reason. New pharmaceutical products will be developed to prevent high-risk individuals from becoming dependent on drugs, alcohol, and perhaps tobacco; substantial progress in this type of prevention is unlikely to be made, however, before the 1990's.

Efficient rehabilitation can, as noted earlier, play a preventive role, so that there is some overlap between these two aspects of health care. In the case of the physically handicapped, the distinction is even more blurred between rehabilitation and treatment; surgery, physiotherapy, the use of prostheses and other artificial devices, modifications of the physical environment, and health education will all be used in the rehabilitation of the physically handicapped.

Surgical methods will become increasingly successful in repairing, compensating, or replacing useless or failing body parts, including the internal organs, limbs, and sense organs, and in repairing nervous and musculo-skeletal damage. In the treatment of nerve injuries, techniques will be developed for by-passing areas of ineffective nerve conduction, followed, by about 1990, by methods for replacing nerves and nerve channels in the spinal cord, while nerve regeneration within the central nervous system may eventually be achieved. Regeneration of striated muscle should be possible by about 1990. Prostheses employing new and more effective materials will be used in repairing joints damaged by injury or disease, while methods may be devised for causing the regeneration of cartilage, obviating the need for prostheses in some types of joint surgery. Effective methods will also be developed for improving the blood supply to ischaemic areas in bones and joints, especially the hip joint.

Physiotherapy will remain an essential sequel to corrective surgery, employing new methods that are developed as further knowledge is acquired about the mechanisms of muscular compensation. Together with surgery and physiotherapy, the use of artificial devices forms the third aspect of a co-ordinated, tripartite approach to rehabilitation, which will be indispensable in the correction or amelioration of many types of physical handicap. Highly functional artificial limbs and other prostheses will be developed through collaboration among orthopaedic surgeons, physiologists, biologists, and electronic engineers. Electronic equipment will be developed to compensate for the loss of innervation and control of limbs and sphincters. Improved types of equipment, designed to compensate for special disabilities, will enable handicapped persons to perform useful jobs, often using remote-control devices. Methods will also be developed for the better compensation of deafness and deaf-mutism, and eventually for blindness, although this is unlikely within the next twenty years.

Besides helping the individual to adapt to his physical environment, attention will turn to planning the environment in order to cater for the special needs of the old and the physically handicapped. A new approach to town planning will evolve, with homes and public buildings constructed to provide easy access, and transportation systems, furniture, and equipment designed to help those with disabilities. This concept of creating a total, functional environment will call for close interdisciplinary collaboration of medicine with the social sciences, ergonomics, engineering, architecture, and town planning. A wider understanding of the problems of the handicapped will be promoted by educational programmes for the public, certain aspects being integrated into the curricula of schools and of trade and professional institutes. Information of this nature will help in gaining society's acceptance of handicapped persons, and ensuring their psycho-social adaptation.

Behaviour therapy for the neuroses and behavioural disorders, aiming to re-condition the individual's responses to psychic stimuli in his environment or to change intrinsic behaviour patterns, as in drug abuse, will form part of both treatment and rehabilitation. These two aspects of health care will thus merge and overlap. The coming years will see the further development of social psychiatry, with group therapy, sometimes at the community level, tending to replace psychoanalysis and other traditional methods of psychotherapy.

How great a burden will the physically and mentally handicapped be to society? It is most likely that their rehabilitation will come to be regarded as a challenge rather than a burden, with the community as a whole striving to re-integrate them as far as their disabilities allow. Meeting the challenge will make increasing economic demands upon the community, on whom the responsibility will fall rather than upon the handicapped person and his family. But what of those who seem to be hopelessly handicapped and cannot be rehabilitated? The grossly damaged, and those with severe genetic defects, who are surviving longer as a result of improved resuscitation techniques and medical care, are already straining the resources of some rehabilitation centres. Since they require a large number of personnel to care for them, not only are these patients non-productive, but by virtue of their incapacity they render others unproductive too. Are they a burden, a challenge, or an obligation? The answer, which depends on the attitudes of society to the handicapped as a whole, will be based on the prevailing ethical, moral, and social values. With regard to those who are severely mentally handicapped, and who cannot 'function' in any useful way, the question of euthanasia will stir up much debate and controversy in the coming decades.

Certain countries already accept the principle that the handicapped should enjoy the same opportunities of education, professional training, and employment as the non-handicapped. This attitude will grow, leading to emphasis on ability rather than disability, and on satisfying particular needs, with a total assessment of each individual and a reluctance to dismiss any case as hopeless. The future approach will be to find out what potential skill and ability the handicapped person possesses which he himself would, realistically, like to develop in order to gain a useful place in society. Educational programmes, supported by publicity campaigns, will aim to create public awareness of the problem of the handicapped and to encourage active involvement in helping them to become integrated into society. Despite these efforts, however, the quality of interpersonal relationships will continue to deteriorate along with the growth of urbanization, with people caring less and less about the problems of others. In a stressful, rapidly changing society, where even healthy people find increasing difficulty in keeping their mental and social equilibrium, how much more difficult will this be for the handicapped.

Rehabilitation of the permanently disabled demands a life-long effort, from school and occasionally university, through the working years, up to and during retirement. While some handicapped persons will live in special homes and villages, the majority will be spread out among the active population rather than remaining grouped together in homogeneous, separate communities; this will facilitate their integration, as well as helping to distribute the moral and economic responsibility. The most severely handicapped will be distributed among communities of other categories of patients also requiring continuous supervision.

The integration of the handicapped into normal activities, alongside healthy people, will extend to their education, social and leisure activities, and work. Sheltered workshops will continue to play a vital role in rehabilitation, providing the link between direct health care, such as surgery, physiotherapy, and speech therapy, and self-sufficiency through active employment. Run under specialized medical supervision, they operate under contracts from business enterprises for types of work that can be performed by handicapped persons. Although run on the lines of a commercial organization, they will in all probability never be economically viable but will be supported by subsidies from governmental and private sources. Vocational guidance will be based on a careful assessment of each individual's handicaps, as well as his capabilities and interests, ensuring suitable training and employment of both the physically and mentally handicapped. Special equipment will be used to compensate for functional disabilities. While this individual approach will require great effort and expense, it will enable nearly all handicapped persons to be productive, and many to be financially self-supporting at least as regards their essential needs. In some countries, hospitals and factories are legally required to employ a quota of physically handicapped persons; an increasing number of jobs will be reserved for them in the future, both through legislation and by promoting interest among leaders of industry in the problems of rehabilitation. This is not altogether a matter of philanthropy, for it is claimed that handicapped persons are stable and devoted workers, who are content to be filling a role compatible with their limitations rather than constantly striving for change or improvement. They often perform repetitive tasks better than fully able workers, and have lower accident rates.

Many handicapped persons will never become productive and will remain the financial responsibility of the community, especially the severely mentally handicapped and an increasing number of the old and disabled. Thousands of others, however, will cease to suffer from the stigma of the crippled person as a being apart, as the boundaries gradually dissolve between normal and pathological, health and disease, ability and disability. The new emancipation of the handicapped, by granting them a sense of fulfilment and independence, will ensure their greater vitality and human dignity.

# 5 | The Physical and Social Environment

Most causes of damage to the environment will not be removed during the next twenty years, but attempts will be made to control them. Until these controls take effect, rising pollution levels and various types of nuisance pose ever-increasing threats to health. As the situation worsens, the need for doctors and other health workers to re-orient themselves towards environmental hygiene is imperative. This shift in emphasis requires changes in the doctor's training and attitudes, which are not easily brought about in a profession that is generally conservative and lagging several years behind the needs of the community. Unless the medical profession adapts quickly enough and undergoes the necessary far-reaching changes, the lead in environmental health may be taken over by sociologists and workers in other disciplines. Taking an optimistic view, the health professions can be seen playing a vital role in the solution of environmental problems, as active participants or advisers in three broad and overlapping areas: preventive medicine, protection and planning of the environment, and attempts to improve the quality of life.

The emphasis is shifting from the sick patient to the healthy individual; from treating disease to striving for the highest possible level of health in terms of physical and mental well-being and social adaptation. The attitudes of the medical profession need to keep pace with these changing perspectives, just as the curricula of medical schools have to be re-oriented. Great research efforts will be devoted to evaluating and preventing the dangers due to air and water pollution, ionizing radiations, noise, and the contamination of food products by additives and pesticides. As the concept of preventive medicine widens, answers will be sought to the problems of failure to adapt to living and working conditions in modern cities, as manifested, for example, by various stress disorders. Occupational medicine will expand rapidly and will gain in importance. Objective criteria will be set by which the 'degree of healthiness' of a particular environment can be measured. Further, ways will be sought of detecting early signs of failure to adapt, manifested by impaired performance in either the working or social context. In urban areas, increasing attention will be given to protection of the nervous system, through teaching health-promoting attitudes to everyday life, better human relations, and the rational use of leisure time.

A new architectural approach is becoming apparent in town planning, with a gradual merging of the functions of the architect and town planner. In future, these functions will be extended, enabling the comprehensive planning not only of towns and cities, but of entire regions or even countries. This integrated approach will enable the urban environment to be planned on a functional basis from the health viewpoint, with advice being sought from the health professions as well as from experts in other disciplines. Provision will be made to protect green areas for recreational and aesthetic purposes, with parks, gardens, and woods easily accessible to all citizens, including mothers and children, the old, and the handicapped. Noise and pollution in residential areas will be reduced by setting up satellite new towns around large cities and by the segregation of industrial areas. By about 1990, a start will be made to provide homes in large urban agglomerations with their own artificial environment, with air conditioning and purification, while improved building methods and materials will further help to reduce noise.

In parallel with these efforts to prevent illness due to a harmful environment, and to construct a better environment through rational planning, steps will be taken to ease the weight of environmental pressures and the tensions of modern life, and to improve the quality of life, through ensuring that working conditions are compatible with physical and mental well-being and by encouraging the effective use of leisure time. Improved opportunities, facilities, and education will be provided for leisure, combined with its organization in a useful and rational way. A 'science of leisure' can be seen evolving over the next decade. Too rational an approach can, of course, kill the therapeutic value of leisure, since the purpose is to escape momentarily from social and economic constraints. Moreover, many people would object to having their leisure time organized by others. Nevertheless, strictly regimented holiday health resorts are proving highly popular, for example, in some of the Baltic republics. Heavily subsidized, they are remarkably inexpensive by Western standards, but are often conducted with a collectivized routine that many would find confining. A typical day begins early, with group morning exercises; breakfast is followed by medical treatment and a prescribed walk on the beach; an hour's rest in the afternoon prepares the holidaymaker for group cultural activities and another prescribed walk in the evening; he eats his yoghurt at 10 p.m. and retires in time for lights out at 11 p.m. The diets prescribed are planned by an institute in Moscow, which also sets the schedule of alternating mudbaths, sulfur immersions, and massages. It would be rash to predict the extent to which such highly organized forms of health-oriented leisure will develop in other countries. What is reasonably certain, however, is that advice and guidance on leisure activities will be given by governmental agencies and the health professions, with facilities provided and often subsidized by public authorities at the local and national levels. Leisure does not, of course, need to be active or organized in order to be beneficial. Health cure resorts will at last be used rationally as centres for relaxation and recuperation from the stresses of life. The final choice regarding the use of leisure will rest with the individual.

Many types of work, including manual work, have positive health value if properly designed and performed in proper dosage. The type of work a man does is already recognized as an essential factor in ensuring his physical and mental well-being, and in the future will be increasingly considered from the health viewpoint. In assessing health and the causes of illness, doctors will pay greater attention to employment; work physiologists and psychologists, specializing in ergonomics, will assist in job planning and job allocation; and a large number of centres will be set up for research on work physiology. Through these efforts, more precise norms and legal standards will be established for working hours and for controlling harmful agents in the working environment.

While many of these developments relate to physical health, increasing attention will be given to the psychological effects of working conditions. There will be a growing demand for longer and more frequent pauses during the working day, longer vacations, and elimination of the sharp division between working and leisure time. Specialists in industrial medicine, as well as work physiologists and psychologists, will work closely with both management and trade unions on questions of working conditions. This interdisciplinary collaboration will seek to ensure that working conditions are not only safe but also have some physical and psychological value, aims which are not merely humanitarian but are manifestly in the interests of greater efficiency and productivity. In industry, it is well documented that boredom, due to tedious and repetitive jobs, can lead to alcoholism and absenteeism, these three evils often reinforcing one another in a vicious circle. The interdisciplinary approach will safeguard the doctor from being pressurized either by malingering employees or by employers. The latter, while not expecting the doctor to set productivity standards, may yet wish him to fill a role comparable to that of an army physician in wartime, in getting his patients back to work as quickly as possible, ensuring their productivity, and enabling them to be discharged when no longer efficient.

As the positive value of manual work becomes further recognized, craftsmanship will flourish during the 1980's as both work and leisure activity, and will find wide application in campaigns to keep people active after retirement.

While the measures outlined above will help man to adapt to an era of unprecedented change and to avoid the harmful effects of a potentially noxious environment, they are merely palliative. They do not strike at the real, underlying causes responsible for the continued deterioration of the environment. For a long time to come, attempts to improve the quality of the environment will be hampered by traditional practices and attitudes. For example, efforts to curtail industrial development will be violently opposed because of the over-riding importance attached to profitability, and the ever-increasing appetite of the consumer society for the fruits of technological progress. A radical attack on the causes of pollution would need far-reaching changes in both industry and the structure of society, entailing enormous costs and difficult political decisions. Consequently, no fundamental solution can be foreseen, in any country, before at least the turn of the century. Not only will industrialization continue to expand apace during the next twenty years, often encroaching on residential areas, but the countryside will be progressively swallowed up by the inexorable process of urban sprawl. The problem of motor vehicles will not be resolved quickly, and for at least the next ten years they will continue to proliferate at an alarming rate, which in some countries is already twice as fast as that of the human population. Cities will be ever more choked with traffic and afflicted with noise and exhaust fumes.

Demographic changes and economic expansion underlie this continuing tendency for the quality of the environment to deteriorate. Here we must make a clear distinction between geographical overcrowding due to the phenomenon of urbanization, and over-population due to a high birth rate, which is essentially a Third World problem. The future population problem in the developed countries will be one of urbanization, carrying with it manifold deleterious effects on the environment, such as air and water pollution, the restriction of recreational facilities, noise, and other nuisances. The future citizen will find himself ever more alone in the anonymous crowd, lonely yet unable to find the physical solitude he craves. Affronted by canned music, television, advertising, and innumerable artificial stimuli, his psyche will be hopelessly unable to adapt, failure to do so causing widespread psychic and psychosomatic disorders. Thus we glimpse, looming over the vast megalopolis of the future, the twin spectres of physical and psychological pollution.

Under the combined influence of demographic and economic expansion, certain industrial zones may have to be abandoned as pollution reaches intolerable levels and protective measures are considered uneconomical. Some industrialized countries have eased their pollution problem through exporting part of their industry to developing countries. This practice may well increase as more developing countries are tempted to accept such importation, aspiring to become industrialized and at the same time believing that pollution does not pose a direct threat. Herein lies a dilemma; if the developed countries apply pollution controls, which are expensive and inevitably add to production costs, the Third World can pour in cheaper goods, and will no doubt object violently if these goods are restricted.

Public concern over the deterioration of the environment, fed by publicity from the mass media plus its all-too-clear manifestations in everyday life, will grow into anxiety and even alarm. Demands will be made for governments to provide comprehensive measures for ensuring a healthy environment. The continued explosion of nuclear devices in the atmosphere, for example, is leading to public outrage and protests. If the practice continues, some people consider that the level of background radiation could reach mutagenic levels by 1990, with a resulting increase in congenital abnormalities and disorders of haematopoiesis. Yet before the highly complex human environment can be subjected to rigorous scientific analysis, a more thorough knowledge of environmental hazards and a more precise concept of medical ecology are needed, through interdisciplinary studies. Over the next few years, environmental control will take the form of short-term measures designed to prevent further deterioration, while awaiting the development of wider and more radical, long-term solutions. A turning point will probably occur about 1980, when control measures take effect and pollution levels begin to fall. The focus will remain on control during the subsequent decade. Measures to control pollution from factories, power plants, motor vehicles, waste disposal, and domestic and other sources will be enforced through legislation. Governments are becoming increasingly aware of the pressing need for such legislation, particularly to control air, water, and noise pollution. As public opinion is further mobilized, the demand for positive action will grow.

By 1980, rigid limits will be set in most countries for noise and pollution levels from motor vehicles and jet aircraft. But not before 1990 will motor vehicles as we know them today be replaced to any large extent by silent and non-polluting forms of transport; later still, the internal combustion engine will be banned from cities. Water pollution will be cut through more effective control of spillage from offshore oil drilling, better regulation of industrial effluents, including thermal discharges, and specific legislation to prohibit pollution by certain toxic substances, such as mercury. Solid wastes, industrial and domestic, will be disposed of efficiently, by incineration and landfill, or re-cycled for further use as a result of improved technology. Better methods will be developed and enforced for the biological treatment of liquid wastes, the elimination of materials not susceptible to such treatment, and the recovery of re-usable industrial wastes. Systematic monitoring of pollution levels, already carried out in certain countries, will be extended on an international scale and combined with an early warning system. A new breakthrough will be the setting up of special research institutes for developing an environmentally favourable technology, where industrial processes can be worked out and tested with a view to preventing environmental pollution at the source. Physicians and biologists will play an important role in this type of research.

The long-term effects of contamination of food products by antibiotics, pesticides, and other chemical pollutants present unknown hazards. They may, for example, lead to future epidemics of hepatic cirrhosis, or degeneration of the central nervous system. As awareness of possible dangers grows, efforts will be made, principally by the Food and Agriculture Organization of the United Nations and the World Health Organization, in collaboration with national governments, to set legal controls over the use of food additives and other contaminants. Although some use of food additives will continue, the food industry will exercise increasing restraint. Maximum permitted levels of application of pesticides will be established, their use being restricted to short periods of time, and new substances will be developed that are less toxic and persistent and have a more selective action. Such is the story of DDT. For years a controversy has raged over the relative hazards due to malaria, on the one hand, and poisoning by this insecticide, on the other.

Legislation to protect the environment will be imposed at the national level and enforced by environmental police under a Ministry of the Environment. In some areas regional agreements will protect rivers and lakes, while international regulations will be laid down to control food contamination and other health hazards. Legislation to limit the increase in industrial pollution will need to be co-ordinated by international agreements, since many forms of pollution spread far beyond the country of origin, while governments will enforce such legislation at the national level. The 1980's will see the proliferation of a multitude of international agreements covering such areas as dumping on the ocean bed, smoke emission levels, and the hazards presented by supersonic air transport. The responsibility for initiating and co-ordinating such agreements will be borne by various international bodies concerned with environmental protection; their influence will grow and their spheres of action will gradually become better defined. To be properly effective, certain wide-scale agreements will need to be universally accepted and to be supervised by the United Nations. Yet universal acceptance of pollution controls presents formidable difficulties, stemming from wide differences in the stage of industrial development reached by different countries throughout the world. In general, the socialist countries of Eastern Europe lag behind the capitalist world, while the Third World has other values and will continue to be concerned with rapid industrialization rather than protection of the environment. Inevitably, the question will arise of imposing sanctions on delinquent nations.

As a result of new legislation, industry will be obliged to carry out research and develop techniques for reducing or eliminating nuisances. This will add to production costs. Incentives may be provided by tax exemptions for non-polluting industries, or through adverse government publicity, leading to loss of markets and financial losses, for those industries that continue to pollute. Intervention of this type could produce quick results. Governments will provide grants for experimental approaches and demonstrations, and loans or subsidies in some cases, but the main burden of increased production costs will be placed on industry, which will pass them on to the consumer as higher prices. The precise method of paying for environmental control in industry will depend on the political system of the country concerned, but in any event the result will be an increased cost to the individual, through the payment of higher taxes or of higher prices for goods consumed. Other sources of financing environmental control will come from the licensing of certain types of industry and the registration of sources of pollution, the fees being diverted directly or indirectly to pay for control measures. Infringement of legislation may be heavily penalized, the fines imposed also helping to defray costs. Governments will assume financial responsibility for large public works that are part of a general environmental plan for a region or urban area, and for controlling nuisances that are not due to a particular industry but to the community as a whole; in some countries, a special environmental tax may be levied for these purposes. Despite massive legislation, it is doubtful whether controls can be thoroughly effective, for two reasons in particular. Firstly, present knowledge of environmental effects is incomplete, and secondly, the rapid development of technology may lead to new forms of pollution as fast as existing ones are controlled.

Attitudes cannot be imposed by law but can be changed through persuasion. The drive to protect the environment will therefore be reinforced by educational and propaganda campaigns, aimed at promoting a consciousness of the problems throughout the entire population and changing the climate of public opinion from the thoughtless attitudes of the consumer society to a high level of responsibility. A variety of educational programmes will be carried out by such bodies as trade unions, employers' federations, schools, and voluntary organizations. Awareness of environmental problems will be promoted in industry through educational programmes for management. Information about environmental protection will be distributed through the mass media and by a variety of audio-visual techniques, and will form part of wider health educational programmes, notably those concerned with preventive medicine. The doctor will participate in all forms of health education as, besides healing the sick, he comes to play a major role in protecting and promoting the well-being of the healthy community.

# 6 | The 'Social Drug'

In 1970, two hundred million prescriptions for psychotropic drugs were dispensed by pharmacists in the USA, an average of one per head of the population. Their cost amounted to approximately a thousand million dollars, equivalent to one-sixth of the total sales turnover for all kinds of pharmaceutical products. Surveys have shown that one adult American out of four takes at least one psychotropic drug regularly, while over half the population use them from time to time. The rate of consumption in the industrialized countries of Europe is comparable; in England, over 15 million prescriptions for barbiturates alone were registered in 1970, to which must be added an unknown number of unrecorded sales.

What is the reason for this enormous consumption of psychotropic drugs? Taken more as a means of defence than for a therapeutic effect, they provide momentary escape or support rather than cure; relief from fatigue, monotony, anguish, frustration, or even the minor anxieties arising in everyday life. Curiously, as the stresses of modern life increase, so is the threshold of tolerance to them becoming progressively lower, so that substances which at one time were taken only for some pressing cause, such as severe insomnia, or profound anxiety, are now ingested almost routinely in anticipation of such minor stresses as starting school or occasional insomnia. These drugs are too often looked on as a panacea, as a chemical screen behind which to escape from the stress of everyday life, as the ultimate recourse in the face of conflict situations. The concept of instant chemical salvation is encouraged to some extent by the pharmaceutical industry and the medical profession. Tranquillizers, it is claimed, help the adolescent to integrate socially, and the child to start school or endure a visit to the dentist. Psychotropic drugs are used to help solve problems of family relationships.

Although psychotropic drugs are, of course, used for valid therapeutic purposes, we have been discussing their use, not in the treatment of illness, but in the alteration of mood or behaviour in response to social circumstances. The term 'social drug' is proposed for agents that are used in this way, as well as for others that may influence social adaptation or behaviour indirectly, such as oral contraceptives or appetite depressants. Many or all of them serve a dual role, as a social drug and a therapeutic agent.

Social drugs are likely to become more numerous and sophisticated in the coming years, with euphoriants, tranquillizers, stimulants, and energizers that are highly effective and specific in their action. Male oral contraceptives will be developed, as well as drugs to induce abortion. Chemical contraceptive agents, affecting the mobility and implantation of the fertilized ovum via chemical transmitters rather than hormones, will act with a minimum of physiological disturbance and low risk; intervention of this nature will blur the distinction between contraception and abortion. New agents will be produced to increase intellectual facilities, stimulate sexuality, reduce obesity, and prevent or treat dependence on drugs, alcohol, and tobacco. Drugs will not be found, however, that slow or prevent the aging process, or even prevent premature senescence, without additional measures being taken from an early age. Products purporting to have a rejuvenating effect will nevertheless be regularly consumed by many in their hopeful quest for perpetual youth.

The importance of anxiety as the major symptom of modern psychopathology is reflected in the growing consumption of tranquillizers. In the USA, their use increased by some 84 % between 1964 and 1970, and now accounts for about 40 % of prescriptions for social drugs of all types. During the same six-year period, the number of prescriptions for hypnotics and stimulants increased by only 17 % and 13 %, respectively. Moreover, while tranquillizers were taken, twenty years ago, mainly by adults of middle or advanced age, their use today, like that of other psychotropic agents, appears to be extending to the younger age groups. Especially disturbing is the growing use of amphetamine derivatives for hyperactive children. In the city of Omaha, Nebraska, it was found recently that, among 62,000 schoolchildren, between 5 % and 10 % were consuming these substances daily. Moreover, in the vast majority of cases they are prescribed, not by a neurologist or psychiatrist, but by a general physician; and not so much to treat the child as to relieve the anxiety of parents or teachers when the child's behaviour does not conform to what they regard as normal.

We are now entering the heyday of social medication. As the environment becomes more complex and the problems of adaptation multiply, the use of psychotropic drugs will soar rapidly. The chemical screen may merely provide a transient escape from problems of social integration or of personal relationships, but there is the danger that it may put off for ever the finding of true solutions to these problems. Between these extremes, such drugs can serve a useful purpose in temporarily modifying the individual's internal environment, as a supplement to the slower and more difficult process of applying requisite social measures. Urged on by the need to resolve his conflicts, together with a search for happiness and an insatiable curiosity to experiment, the future citizen will consume ever-greater amounts of these substances, which within a decade will come to be regarded as a necessary part of modern life. This is the position occupied for years by tea, coffee, and alcoholic beverages, the psychotropic ingredients of which are, however, relatively harmless. In the absence of definitive social solutions, doctors will not only condone the use of psychotropic drugs as a temporary and supportive measure, but will acquiesce in prescribing them as a panacea. As their consumption rises they will cause an increasing amount of harm through their toxic effects, but it will be some years before their dangers come to be widely recognized and controlled.

With growing public demand, governments will feel obliged to make social drugs more easily available and to ensure their low cost. While most will be available only on prescription, others, including marijuana, will be freely on sale. As the annual cost of such medication continues to mount rapidly, the question of which social drugs, if any, should be paid for out of the national health budget will stimulate much controversy. The effectiveness and specificity of psychotropic drugs will be enhanced as a result of research into the biochemical basis of anxiety, depression, and emotional disorders. Progress will also be made in reducing or eliminating certain adverse reactions, through the development of new products and the determination of precise indications and dosages. As society, encouraged by new developments such as these, becomes increasingly permissive towards the use of social drugs, detailed studies will be undertaken of the relationship between social medication and an ethic of behaviour.

The permissive attitude will change, however, once certain dangers arising from the massive use of psychotropic drugs become manifest. Drug-induced mental disturbances, for example, leading to further medication, can set up a vicious circle; this has already been observed in France. These drugs may be a danger spot in future medical care unless action is taken in time to prevent large-scale catastrophes. A reaction against their use can therefore be envisaged on the part of health authorities, encouraged by pressure from social groups and leading to the introduction of strict controls over psychotropic drugs. Campaigns will also be launched to inform the public of the dangers involved.

Another type of danger will largely be responsible for turning the tide of public feeling against the use of these substances. Drugs which modify the psychological state are capable of destroying the integrity of the individual, while replacing it perhaps with an illusion of freedom. The way is thus open to tyranny, or at least to an occult form of social manipulation, should a small number of people ever be in a position to control the pharmacological conditioning of a community or an entire population. Besides freedom, equality will be called into question with the development of drugs to increase intellectual ability. Who will be given them, and why? Can they, too, be misused for political ends? Public reaction against psychotropic drugs will be strengthened, moreover, by a growing realization that many of their apparent benefits are illusory, and that their use is a confession of failure both by the individual and by society. Doctors, becoming oriented towards community care and concern for the total human environment, will recognize their moral and professional duty to encourage this trend. From attempting, by artificial means, to change the individual in accordance with the expectations of society, efforts will thus be directed with renewed vigour to adapting the social environment to the needs of the individual.

With the imposing of strict controls, a highly profitable black market in psychotropic drugs will no doubt spring up, associated with problems of drug abuse among the minority of people who continue to consume them illegally. Public authorities and social groups will then try, unsuccessfully, to stamp out their illicit use. Will this be followed by a return to liberalization? Quite conceivably, the situation could come full circle through successive phases – drugs being freely available, government-imposed restrictions, illegal use, and a further move towards liberalization. Psychotropic drugs could thus follow the pattern of alcohol consumption in the USA before, during, and after Prohibition.

# 7 | The Concept of Health

We are told, by one of today's foremost if more pessimistic futurologists, that the world may face 80 possible crises by 1985. Doomwatchers predict that our globe may be over-populated, over-polluted, over-urbanized, and overcome by race conflicts, to name only a few disasters in store. Hope of averting these dangers lies in new social attitudes and a growing concern for the quality of life, which are replacing blind faith in technological progress. As this new emphasis reflects the changing concept of health, the views of the medical profession are likely to have an increasingly significant impact on governmental schemes for social prophylaxis.

As the emphasis shifts from the curing of disease to the maintenance of health, prevention and early detection will grow in importance as part of a continuum of services that includes diagnosis, treatment, rehabilitation, and health education. With the development of mass screening programmes to detect predisposition to disease and to identify high-risk cases, the concept of subclinical pathology will assume great significance within the next few years. By 1980, evaluation of the risk in these cases by computers will be a familiar concept to doctors, enabling them to apply prophylactic measures where necessary. In the case of clinical disease, too much significance is often attached to advances made in the treatment of rare or difficult conditions; the more spectacular a new development, the more its importance is exaggerated. However, since human beings twenty years from now will still suffer from sore throats, fractures, hernias, and peptic ulcers, it would be erroneous to think that the cost of prestigious new developments will be allowed to detract from the treatment of common ailments.

In both the capitalist and socialist worlds, the concept of mental illness will be broadened to include disorders arising from the so-called 'sick society', including behavioural disturbances and difficulties of interpersonal relationships. Intensive sociological studies to define and diagnose the social pathology that is responsible, combined with a growing emphasis on community health, will lead to progressive socio-political changes. The medical profession, although traditionally conservative, will gradually adapt its role in order to help bring about these changes. While the mental health services deal increasingly with group problems, for example intra-family conflicts, health care of the individual will become ever more concerned with psychosomatic illness, behavioural disorders, and other difficulties of adaptation to life, as well as with organic disease.

The widening concept of mental health to embrace physical, intellectual, and emotional behaviour will lead to the growth of experimental psychology and an expanding technology of behaviour. School learning difficulties and the development of new teaching methods will enter the domain of medicine, as will the treatment of minor aggressions that are now regarded as part of normal behaviour. Tomorrow's doctors will not only treat medical problems arising from behavioural disorders, but will advise on solutions of their underlying causes based on sociology and the behavioural sciences.

The ethical problems that arise from new drugs or other methods of influencing the mind have begun to arouse concern, in particular regarding a future technology of behaviour control that might threaten personal liberty. Modern methods make it possible to exact individual conformity with greater reliability and less resistance than ever before. Singly or in combination, psychological conditioning techniques, drugs, and neurosurgical methods for controlling brain functions electrically or chemically, via implantations, are the most important among a host of methods which will be available to manipulate mood, emotion, and desire so precisely that large areas of behaviour can be removed from the individual's control and placed under that of others. Most of these controls will presumably be in the hands of doctors, whose efforts will be directed to curing psychosis, aggression, obesity, and other behaviour-related disorders. Some, however, will surely become available to officials concerned with law enforcement for use on behalf of society, whether the individual likes it or not; and the danger is that the controlled individual can be made to like it. The development of control methods which eliminate personal freedom, while leaving people with the feeling they are free, may sound ideal from a correctional or rehabilitation standpoint, but it undermines conventional morality on which democracy is based.

In addition to this awesome enlargement of medical potential, the changing concept of health has less terrifying aspects. The conventional view of health as the absence of disease or infirmity is being replaced by a positive concept, one of health as good functional performance within a given frame of reference that takes into account physical and psychological impediments. As the emphasis shifts to abilities rather than disabilities, ways will be developed of quantifying functional well-being, for example in terms of capacity for work or social integration. In both children and adults, the concept of health will include physical fitness and attempts to delay the aging process, while in the elderly it will be related to ensuring the maximum prolongation of an independent life, helped by adequate social relationships and community services. At present it is not so much a question of adding years to the life expectancy as of preserving useful function for as many years as possible. Young people's concept of health, while centred mainly on freedom from injury and disease, is turning more to the need for personal development, self-fulfilment, and the ability to enjoy life. Their attempts to impress authorities with the need for social changes, however, are frustrated by their ignorance and lack of adequate guidance. Although the voice of youth will hardly be a decisive influence, health workers will in the future encourage activities that help people to feel their lives are meaningful even though their health is impaired. As health becomes synonymous with well-being, types of treatment that are today a luxury will become the health right of every individual, with cosmetic care of the teeth, skin, and hair freely available. Research in dermatology will result in new medicines and surgical procedures that help the aged to retain a youthful appearance. With the growing effort to slow down the aging process and avert degenerative diseases, few conditions of old age will be viewed as inevitable causes of decline and death. The amount of chronic disease will nevertheless increase as a result of an aging population, leading to greater emphasis on long-term and geriatric care.

As the costs of medical care mount, the community will demand increasing rights over the health of the individual, and in return will share the responsibility for his well-being. The right to health will be viewed rather like the right to freedom; just as one cannot consider that a man is truly free while his neighbour is in chains, neither will he be regarded as completely healthy while others around him are sick. Demands for health care are influenced by health education and by concepts of well-being and the right to health; the point at which people seek help thus depends on their notions of what is normal, tolerable, curable, and desirable. Demands tend to increase as long as means are available for satisfying them, while the development of new methods of care and new health services evoke further demands. The additional need for treatment arising from mass screening programmes, for example, will rapidly overwhelm the available resources, and it will take decades before such programmes lead to a significant drop in the amount of disease. Health costs, therefore, far from being self-limiting, will tend to augment in snowball fashion. Studies already completed or under way on the factors that influence people in their use of health care services need to be greatly expanded.

Although health does not have a measurable value for the individual, it does have a budget for the community. Ever-rising costs will oblige health authorities to apply cost-benefit analysis to all aspects of health care, as part of the decision-making process in allocating limited resources. If the benefits of a rising level of health are measured in terms of national productivity, a point of diminishing returns is reached soon after the basic health needs of the population are satisfied. This criterion is heavily biased against the aged, who are largely unproductive and yet whose health needs are the greatest. The aged, however, are unlikely to be the victims of discrimination. On the contrary, since they form a growing percentage of the electorate their rising clamour for treatment, requiring a far greater share of national health resources, may amount to no less than a 'tyranny' of the aged. Final decisions among competing programmes will be made in the political arena, with cost-benefit analysis merely an economic tool for the decision maker. Politically, health care occupies a place of growing importance and is competing for priority with the production of wealth; the next decade will witness a conflict between the demands of production and the requirements of life.

With medicine becoming oriented to social and community concepts, the doctor needs to understand those environmental factors that cause physical, mental, and emotional disability and that influence social adaptation. He will feel impelled to abandon his traditional role of observer by volunteering constructive criticism of social conditions from the health viewpoint. As his horizons spread and as health concepts are incorporated into social, cultural, educational, and economic programmes, the doctor will be called upon for advice and co-operation in diverse fields of direct or indirect health interest. Along with scientists in various disciplines related to medicine, he will increasingly give advice on, for example, housing, town and country planning, working conditions, transport, and legislation. Concern for hygiene is giving way to the concept of healthiness, as part of total environmental planning whether applied to a building, district, town, area, or entire country. While medicine reaches out into other disciplines, so will architects, town planners, engineers, sociologists, and others be accorded a legitimate role in promoting health.

The concept of well-being implies the satisfaction of subjective and objective needs, leading to a state of inner equilibrium and a harmonious rapport with the outside world. It requires a balance between body and mind, between material and spiritual needs, between the individual and his physical and social environment, and the reconciling of his aspirations with those of the community. Conflicting notions of well-being underlie the present revolt by young people against the Establishment, which may not only affect the medical profession but may also lead to profound changes in the structure and moral values of Western civilization. What are the nature and causes of this rebellion? Firstly, it is a rejection by the younger generation of the consumer society, which to them represents human exploitation, wastage, damage to the environment, excessive concern for profit, and a demand for conformity. Secondly, the young person is trying to adapt his life-style in such a way as to satisfy his own concept of well-being.

Society may disintegrate as youth's refusal to collaborate with the existing social system becomes more widespread, and as so-called behavioural disorders increase. Family and religion are tending to be replaced by the concept of social groups, which reject conventional standards of regular employment, shelter, dress, diet, sexual behaviour, and family relationships. As these standards have evolved in close relationship with health, their abandonment is fraught with many direct health dangers such as malnutrition, venereal diseases, and drug abuse. Traditional moral values are being questioned in the search for a new social order. Since morality is a changeable concept, views and behaviour that are today regarded as anti-Establishment may tomorrow be generally accepted. Just as certain types of sexual behaviour, for example, have come to be tolerated in recent years, so may today's confrontation of the martini-drinkers with the pot-smokers lead, by a similar process, to a re-appraisal of the use of social drugs. As quickly as unconventional views become assimilated into society's norms, they are replaced by other manifestations of non-conformity and protest. The questioning of moral values is thus a never-ending process, which may be looked on as a driving force for progress, whether for good or evil, through bringing about changes in those values. With the conscience of youth goading society into a moral self-examination, the veil of hypocrisy is slowly being lifted from Western behaviour. In future, the Establishment will be called upon to justify its actions and to explain its value judgements.

The health professions, no longer content merely to treat symptoms, such as drug abuse and other behavioural disorders, will feel duty-bound to define the underlying causes of this social ferment and to participate in radical solutions. They will seek new objectives, appropriate to the changing needs of society. As the attack on the Establishment is based largely on left-wing concepts, it will tend to have a socializing influence on the medical profession, helping to reduce the doctor's social status as well as the traditional aura surrounding the doctor-patient relationship. The health care of those who opt out of society may become so costly as to influence political, social, and moral attitudes. In coping with the youthful rebellion, therefore, where a choice lies between hospital or prison, medicine or the law, it could well be politicians rather than the health professions who dictate the policies and provide the means for healing the sick society. The question then, is whether doctors will serve as mere technicians in the service of the State.

# Organization of Health Care

# 8 | Health Professions

*The Doctor*

The increasing demands for health care can be met most economically by using doctors more efficiently, while training larger numbers of other health personnel to a lower level of professional competence. As individual practice gives way to the concept of teamwork, the doctor will be relieved by others of minor clinical tasks, burdensome administrative duties, and dealing with social problems in which he is not expert, while remaining the key figure in the health care system with final responsibility for making critical decisions. At the same time he will be able to call upon his medical and non-medical colleagues for the exchange of information, opinions, and advice. The general practitioner, by tradition friend, confessor, and counsellor to his patients, is being swiftly transformed into the leader of, or partner in, a health team that dispenses a more efficient, if less folksy, style of medicine. Group practice will in future allow him more time to listen to and evaluate his patients' problems and will provide him with more effective means for planning and organizing the strategy for dealing with them. Teamwork will also ensure more efficient utilization of the skills of hospital specialists, who are trained to ever-higher levels of expertise in increasingly narrow fields.

How well does the doctor's training equip him for his future role? The objectives of medical training today are unclear, not only to students and doctors but even to the majority of teachers, with the result that much of the knowledge imparted to the medical student is irrelevant to the problems he will meet in everyday practice. While the information the student receives does keep pace with medical progress, its content hardly allows for the changing needs of the community and the changing concept of health. Consequently, medical training produces doctors who are ill-adapted to present needs; even worse, they may be inadaptable to future requirements owing to the rapidity with which new knowledge is accumulating and with which society, its values, and its attitudes are evolving.

Medical training in future will become oriented more towards defined objectives. As a result, its duration will be shortened. This trend will be encouraged by the high cost of medical education and the need to produce more doctors, and helped by more efficient teaching using audio-visual methods. Basic sciences may well be reduced in the curriculum, with greater emphasis on epidemiology, preventive medicine, rehabilitation, and geriatrics. New subjects to be introduced will include sociology, psychology, and economics, while general practice, already taught in some medical schools, will gain wide recognition as a specialty. In future, not only will the student's knowledge, skills, and attitudes be assessed but his teachers and training curriculum will periodically be evaluated.

At the postgraduate level, greater emphasis will be placed on preparing the doctor for a particular specialty. This training period will be shortened and more goal-oriented as specialties grow in number and become narrower in scope. Continuing postgraduate education, on the other hand, will last throughout the doctor's entire career, the need for it growing ever greater in order to keep pace with the rapid development of medical science and technology. In future it could be made a condition for retaining a licence to practise, the amount of training required per year depending on the doctor's specialty. The title of specialist may be given for a limited period and only renewed if the requisite amount of further training has been received. Refresher courses and seminars will be provided in hospitals, health centres, and model group practices.

As the one-to-one relationship of single practice, so characteristic of medical care in the past, diminishes, it may sometimes appear to the patient that he is being treated by non-medical personnel and machines and that he has virtually lost touch with the doctor. The medical profession will make strenuous efforts to preserve the essential ingredients of the traditional relationship. Delegation of work to others and the use of automation, by relieving the doctor of many time-consuming and routine chores, will enable him to give his patients more careful and individual attention; thus the human element may actually be enhanced. This applies especially to the general practitioner and the general physician. In the large hospitals, doctors engaged in a narrow field of specialization, and highly specialized allied health personnel, will be ever more detached from the personal element of health care, which will be provided mainly by the lower echelons of health workers. A few doctors will remain in private practice in most countries and there will always be some people who choose to buy an hour of their time, paying for it themselves or through private health insurance schemes.

Governments, assuming greater responsibility for financing the health services, will try to exercise more control in order to ensure their efficiency and economy. While most doctors will eventually not object to being salaried employees of a socialized health service, they will strenuously resist any attempt to turn them into agents of the State; governments will be aware of the need to respect professional freedom in order to ensure high standards of care. Although public respect for medical science and technology and for the medical profession is increasing, the authority and status of the individual doctor are tending to decline. Within a decade they could be no greater than those of experts in other fields.

## Allied Health Personnel

Those workers who complement the doctor's activities within the health services comprise the allied health professions. New categories are being created as the growing complexity of medicine demands ever-greater specialization and as needs and gaps in the existing system become apparent. Some of them assume tasks that were formerly assigned exclusively to the doctor, and which may lie outside their legal competence. With increasing diversity, the responsibility and skills required of each category of personnel must be more clearly defined, and strict regulations imposed to govern their professional activity and to ensure that the doctor retains ultimate authority and responsibility. Alongside the medical and allied health professions, a variety of non-medical workers, from teachers and town planners to electronic engineers and systems analysts, will play an indirect role in health promotion as the concept of health care widens. Schoolteachers, for example, will be given the task of detecting visual, auditory, and psychological problems, especially those related to reading and learning difficulties and behavioural disorders.

The nurse, who is being trained to carry out a widening variety of technical and administrative procedures, will need to guard against the danger of losing or neglecting those skills in personal care that make her unique and indispensable. Within a decade nursing will no longer be a unified profession, since it will in effect embrace a number of different professions, for example those of intensive care technician, psychiatric worker, and public health nurse, each requiring different skills. The nursing profession will thus be obliged to undergo radical changes, diversifying into specialized categories adapted to future needs. Either it will meet this challenge, through a drastic re-orientation of skills and training, or certain functions will be taken over by another category of health profession, the medical assistant.

The nurse's training, like that of the doctor, will be more goal-oriented. Nurses helping in mass detection campaigns or working in geriatric facilities may require only one year of training, whereas three or four years will be needed for specialist nurses in health centres and major hospitals. Specialization will be structured according to tasks and category of patients, rather than, as at present, to various aspects of nursing, such as clinical nursing, teaching, or administration.

The nurse will take over an increasing number of tasks from the doctor, referring the patient to him or to specialized clinics when difficulties arise; therapy nurses, for example, will be responsible for the continuous treatment of selected groups of patients with hypertension, diabetes, chronic nephritis, and other conditions. She will in turn be relieved of some tasks by nursing auxiliaries. As the doctor's collaborator in the health team rather than as a subordinate carrying out his instructions, it is the nurse who will be mainly responsible for preserving human contact with patients whether in the hospital, health centre, or group practice. She will also share the doctor's co-ordinating role in the health team. Outside health facilities, certain nurses will achieve a large measure of independence. The nurse-midwife will be responsible for routine prenatal and postpartum care, supervision during labour, and family and pre-marital counselling. Some nurses may be trained as paediatric assistants responsible for well baby care, immunizations, routine health examinations, screening tests of hearing and vision, and routine home visits. The home care nurse, with a training in the social sciences, will be even more important than the doctor in providing continuing geriatric care. Home care auxiliaries, with a basic training of only a few days or weeks, will provide elementary care under the supervision of the nurse and the doctor. Public health nurses will be active in preventive medicine, helping to carry out health evaluations and to provide health education.

The tremendous shortage of doctors in some regions has led to the creation of a new allied health profession, that of the medical assistant — also known as the medical aid, physician assistant, or feldsher, and by a variety of other synonyms. His training and responsibility, intermediate between those of the doctor and the present-day nurse, enable him to carry out simple diagnosis and treatment, working more or less independently but under medical supervision. This role, as well as a variety of skilled tasks in health centres, hospitals, and the home, could be filled equally well by medical assistants or by specially trained nurses. Who assumes responsibility in the coming decades will depend on whether the nursing profession can adapt sufficiently and quickly enough to meet the challenge.

Other allied health personnel with a clinical role are those providing various kinds of therapy, for example the physiotherapist, occupational therapist, speech therapist, and dental therapist. Owing to the wide range of functions performed by the polyvalent physiotherapist, there will be less workers of this type, since many will specialize in occupational therapy, rehabilitation, ergotherapy, or speech therapy. Occupational therapy and rehabilitation will develop greatly under the pressure of an aging population and an increasing number of road accident victims and physically handicapped persons. A greater number of speech therapists will be needed as a result of developments in pedagogy, such as the growing emphasis on the correction of learning difficulties in children. Another category of allied health personnel, the dental therapist, has recently been introduced in South Australia, although such dental auxiliaries have existed in New Zealand for some 50 years. In only two years, these young women are trained to treat dental caries in schoolchildren at a standard that compares favourably with that of dental graduates, and to provide dental education through the teaching of healthy dietary habits and oral hygiene.

In non-clinical fields a large number of new allied health professions will appear. Hospital hygienists will take over from bacteriologists the responsibility for controlling infections and cross-infections. Specialized technicians will be employed to maintain and operate the increasingly complex and sophisticated medical equipment in hospitals and diagnostic centres. The medical engineer concerned with developing limb and other prostheses for the physically handicapped must have a knowledge of engineering, electronics, and medicine; this specialty will make enormous strides, forming an invaluable part of the rehabilitation effort. Health education, already a new profession in some countries, will expand rapidly. Leisure advisers, another new profession, will give guidance on physical culture, sport, and other health-promoting uses of leisure time.

Training in certain allied health professions, for example physiotherapy and pharmacy, is now so long and expensive that these groups are faced by a problem that confronted the medical profession some decades ago; it is uneconomical for them to perform certain tasks that can be delegated to less qualified persons. The need for less highly trained assistants to some allied health personnel will soon be acutely felt. However, assistants of this type will face an initial struggle before doctors and patients accept them as an important part of the health services.

It is sometimes questioned whether the profession of pharmacist will disappear, or at least be radically transformed. It has changed considerably in the past; we no longer need the skilled measurer of ingredients and compounder of medicines who flourished in individual practice until some twenty years ago. What of the future? With the explosive development of the number, potency, and use of therapeutic agents, the most conspicuous emerging need is for a new type of allied health professional who is expert in clinical pharmacology and who can handle and distribute these substances safely and effectively. The role of the pharmacist must change accordingly, and will be linked to alterations in the system of drug distribution and the nature of drug prescribing. With increasing governmental control over the pharmaceutical industry, fewer brands of the same drug will be produced and most of the essential ones will be prescribed by their generic names. As part of the attempt to reduce prices, profit margins of producers and distributors will be controlled and certain forms of advertising, for example through free samples for doctors, minimized or abolished. As medicines tend increasingly to become a commodity of the consumer society, attempts will be made to rationalize their use by doctors and the public. They will be dispensed through government-controlled drug distribution centres, some of which will be located in hospitals or health centres. The pharmacist will fill a new role as manager of such a centre rather than as the owner of a private pharmacy. His training will make him more of a pharmacologist than a commercial dispenser of prescribed drugs and purveyor of non-prescription medicines. He will be called upon to advise doctors and will carry the legal responsibility for the dispensing of drugs by the distribution centre. His new role will lead to a closer and more equal relationship with the medical profession. The traditional pharmacist will survive, however, for the sale of non-prescription medicines, cosmetics, toiletries, and health foods.

Allied health personnel will be trained and employed in keeping with governmental guidelines for health teams, the allocation of tasks and the need to create new categories being brought under periodic review. The duration of training will vary; for some specialties it could comprise two years of liberal arts or general science training, and two years of training in a specialty, followed by a year of in-service training. It will be partly integrated into medical schools. In some countries, for example Australia, special colleges for the allied health professions are being developed within colleges of advanced education, for the training of physiotherapists, pharmacists, medical social workers, radiographers, and laboratory technicians. Nursing training is likely to become more closely linked to these colleges. At the lower levels, training may be provided by technical colleges and voluntary organizations. Continuing postgraduate education will be systematic, permanent, and perhaps obligatory for all types of personnel through regular refresher courses, while advancement up the careers ladder will be possible as a result of added specialty and in-service training. Far more young people will be attracted to the allied health professions over the next ten or twenty years as the status and career prospects improve.

The expansion of the allied health professions carries political implications. As a professional body without a fundamental philosophy or a tradition of independence they could be easy prey to over-zealous governmental control, far more so than the medical profession, which, even though state-employed and salaried, will always regard itself as an elite corps of individualists.

Teamwork in the health services cannot be taken for granted, owing to the increasing number and diversity of personnel. Failure of co-operation between all grades and specialties, particularly between doctors and nurses, could undermine the entire system of health care. Compounding the problem is the fact that the doctor's training, and the present structure of medical practice, tend to make him egoistic and individualistic; orienting the doctor towards the team concept must be a priority concern of medical schools and teaching hospitals, which first have to radically change their own mentality and attitudes. Allied health personnel will acquire some notions of teamwork at all stages of their training and through their work, but this is not enough; co-operation will also be specifically taught, as in 'task force' training in graduate town planning schools, where architects, town planners, landscape architects, economists, and sociologists work together. This type of training, which includes group and interpersonal psychology, will lay the foundation for a new and more flexible type of organization to replace the rigid, hierarchical structure of existing health services.

# 9 | Health Services

Most hospitals that will be operating in twenty years' time are already built or in the planning stage. Many will be obsolescent before they open their doors. In attempts to rationalize planning according to future needs, most countries will have socialized their health services to a greater or lesser extent by 1980, although many will also retain a private sector. Even the USA, where most doctors will almost certainly remain self-employed, may well have a universal health care financing programme with substantial governmental control over its organization and cost. The system adopted will often be a compromise between the interests of the consumers and providers of health care. International co-operation in the field of health, expanding enormously over the coming decades, will help to optimize health care systems and will lead to some degree of uniformity in the medical services of different countries.

As demands for hospital care continue to increase, supply and demand, far from being self-limiting, reinforce one another in a rising spiral, with the result that needs are growing or being recognized more rapidly than are the means of satisfying them. This problem will be aggravated in the future by the aging of the population. Although persons over the age of 65 years now constitute only about one-eighth of the total population, they account for some 40 % of hospital bed requirements, or over 50 % if one includes homes and long-term care facilities for the aged. They spend, on average, four times as many days in hospital per year as the population as a whole. The aging population will influence hospital morbidity patterns towards a predominance of chronic diseases, requiring more nursing than medical care. There could, as a result, be a relative shortage of personnel to provide for the patient's daily bedside needs. Improved ambulatory services will merely have the effect of delaying hospital admission until patients are older and their condition more severe. The most frequent answer to the growing demand for hospital care is to provide more beds. Logical as this may appear, it tends to encourage hospitalization that might be avoided by remedies which are cheaper and more effective, albeit less spectacular. Owing to budgetary competition between hospital and ambulatory care, and between health and other public services such as education, housing, social security, and leisure facilities, planning of hospitals and health services by objectives and systems analysis is an urgent requirement. It could lead to substantial changes in the provision of health care, with greater rationalization and efficiency.

Health services will be organized on a regional basis. The large hospital or university medical centre will form the hub of the system, in close association with the regional health centre. Further outward at the district level, in a progressively decentralized hierarchy, will be the district general hospitals, surrounded by various types of facility including polyclinics, group practices, general day hospitals, preventive medicine and health information centres, drug distribution centres, and special facilities for mental illness, geriatrics, and rehabilitation. At the periphery of the health services, home care provided by allied health personnel will be augmented where necessary by specially equipped mobile units. The use of mobile coronary care units has been introduced in recent years in many countries and is expanding; they can considerably reduce hospital mortality rates by providing intensive care almost immediately after the onset of myocardial infarction. The more highly specialized the services, the larger will be the population served, while simpler forms of care will be decentralized as much as possible. The high cost of acute hospital treatment will demand that patients be admitted only when ambulatory care or treatment in other, less specialized facilities would not suffice. These alternatives must be developed if comprehensive health care is to be feasible for the entire population. As health comes to be regarded as a community responsibility, health authorities may eventually, in some countries, take the initiative in ensuring that needs are properly satisfied. Health services will thus form a highly integrated network, providing a continuum of care from prevention and diagnosis to treatment and rehabilitation. A new type of administrator will be needed, not only in large health facilities but for co-ordinating the various links in health care. He should ideally be a doctor, as well as being qualified in economics and administration.

The large hospital will be reserved for severe cases and for difficult diagnostic and therapeutic problems requiring highly specialized personnel or complex and expensive equipment. Conversely, simpler cases will be channelled to facilities at a more peripheral level. As a result it will be possible to reduce the size of some hospitals, thereby helping to avoid many difficulties due to the agglomeration of personnel, equipment, and services in a large, polyvalent hospital complex. A modular type of construction will be introduced to allow a certain flexibility, permitting the physical structure to be re-organized to accommodate new types of service and equipment. Each hospital department will be subdivided into units providing intensive, intermediate, and minimal care, with a final rehabilitation unit.

The regional health centre will provide highly efficient ambulatory care by health teams using sophisticated equipment and automated methods of investigation. Polyclinics will supply diagnostic services at the district level, obviating the need for the general practitioner to refer ambulant patients to the regional health centre. Employing general and specialist physicians and allied health personnel, these polyclinics will provide specialized services for various types of investigation. Hostel-type accommodation will enable patients to stay for a few days when necessary.

While there will be a need for more geriatric beds, old-age homes may disappear entirely in their traditional form. The high-mortality terminal institution is an anachronism in view of the technical, social, and financial means that are becoming available for improving the lives of the elderly. It seems unlikely that the need for geriatric beds can be reduced through families taking over the care of their old folk, since families are becoming more dispersed and the psychological gap between the generations is widening.

Apart from a few remaining single-handed general practitioners, home visits will no longer be made by the doctor but by allied health personnel, some of whom will become responsible for making a preliminary diagnosis or for rehabilitation. A special transportation system will be developed for carrying the sick to the district or regional hospital and, when necessary, for taking ambulant patients to their local group practice or regional health centre. Sparsely populated rural areas are likely to be served by small planes or helicopters bringing the patient to the regional health facility. While small mobile hospitals to serve rural areas are a possibility, an efficient transportation service would be a more practical solution.

In some countries, the lack of a national planning policy for the health services has been tacitly accepted up to the present. Within the next decade or two, a new approach to planning will become imperative if an efficient and well co-ordinated complex of health care services is to be created, with integration of preventive, therapeutic, and rehabilitation facilities. In response to the demands of a better informed public for more efficient health programmes, governments will experiment in new systems of health care, as a result of which health services in different countries may develop along different lines. The universal basic requirement is to establish objectives through epidemiological forecasting of the population's future health needs. This has not yet been carried out with complete success anywhere in the world, although health planning needs in the USSR have been forecast with considerable accuracy. Once future needs have been assessed, an interdisciplinary approach to planning will be indispensable. Mixed consultative committees will be set up which include doctors, pharmacists, biologists, sociologists, lawyers, economists, and specialists in psychology, pedagogy, and information techniques. They will consider ethical, economic, and social problems posed by scientific developments; recommend modifications of existing legislation; and advise on technical and budgetary priorities. Health planning, like planning in other areas, is a question of achieving policy objectives using available resources in the most rational way; this requires modern management techniques such as operational research, analytical and predictive management, and dynamic programming. Policy objectives will be based on budgetary and socio-economic decisions, while manpower, services, and equipment need to be considered in terms of supply and demand, production and consumption, efficiency and market organization. Contrary to what is often argued, efficiency is not incompatible with humanitarian aims.

National planning will be centralized, with inputs and feedback from the regional and district levels. Services, on the other hand, will be decentralized, with regional and local bodies assuming greater management and financial responsibility. The system will be organized to facilitate the two-way flow of patients, from the general practitioner inwards to the health centre and the regional hospital, and outwards from the regional facility to the group practice. The regional hospital, at the hub of the system, will have overall responsibility for the quality of all aspects of health care in the region, including preventive medicine, rehabilitation, and health education.

# 10 | Information

## *Information for the Health Professions*

Within a decade or two the doctor will keep abreast of developments in his profession by clipping in a video-cassette, or tuning in to special television programmes. More important still, he will have instant access by telephone or car radio to his regional information centre, which will answer his queries on any medical subject and provide specific data for use in diagnosing and treating his patients, including their case histories. These new means of communication will help to cope with the information explosion and will lead to more efficient health care. In medicine, as in other areas, the use of computers is becoming ever more widespread and essential for effective communication. In the USA, electronic data processing expenditure by business and industry is expected to show a four- or five-fold increase between 1970 and 1980, the rapid expansion in the consumption of information being encouraged by the falling cost of transmitting, storing, and processing each unit. While the written medium serves a useful function in carrying news and as a forum for discussion, it is no longer adequate when specific information is being sought. Medical journals, discussions, and seminars will in future be supplemented to an ever-greater extent by a new technology using electronic data processing and audio-visual techniques.

Computerized regional information centres will be set up, either as separate facilities or as departments of information within regional hospitals and university medical centres. They will provide, on request, current information on virtually all medical subjects; they will answer queries relating to diagnostic and therapeutic problems, by correlating given symptoms with diseases and suggesting standard treatment, including data on contra-indications and adverse reactions to any drugs that are recommended; they will provide doctors with information on individual patients from the patient data bank; and they will act as a pharmaceutical reference service, giving information on indications, contra-indications, and adverse reactions. The doctor will be able to dial a number and receive immediately the information he needs, by telephone, videophone, or individual car radio. Computer terminals will also link the information centre to health centres, polyclinics, and group practices. Material will be fed to the centre from a variety of sources, mainly university medical centres and international organizations, for example the World Health Organization, with specialists and interdisciplinary teams helping in its selection. Summaries, reviews, and translations will be made where appropriate. A central body will be set up by the universities and the medical profession to co-ordinate information centres at the national level, the amount of governmental control or participation depending on the political structure of the health services.

Computerized patient data banks at the regional information centre will make storage and retrieval far easier and quicker than using conventional medical dossiers. As well as being supplied to doctors for use in health care, these data will provide the material for a statistical reporting system, which may develop, for example, as a by-product of a comprehensive national insurance programme. They will also be used in statistical and epidemiological research, being of particular value in prospective studies. However, many fundamental ethical and medico-statistical problems remain to be solved before the use of data banks for statistical purposes becomes a practical proposition. They can only be used effectively in this way, moreover, once data is stored on the entire population of the region covered by the information centre, probably not until the mid-1980's. Subsequently, data on population groups will be exchanged on an inter-regional and international basis. A co-ordinating, central statistical office will be maintained at the national level. The system may be developed to the point where all health data on the entire population is recorded from birth to death. A computerized, United Nations world information centre for health and environmental data can be envisaged, along the lines of the World Health Organization's research centre for international monitoring of adverse reactions to drugs.

Patient data banks will come to be regarded as indispensable, since they are the only way of dealing scientifically, economically, and efficiently with the enormous mass of information arising from, and needed in, daily medical practice. Yet serious ethical and practical problems arise from the need to safeguard the confidentiality of a vast amount of personal health data. Many personnel involved in handling the data will not, like the doctor, be bound by obligations of professional secrecy. Socialized health services, in which such a system could be of greatest value, must guard against a lack of sensitivity to the rights and feelings of the individual. Will the patient be told, or asked to give his consent, when information about him is fed into the computer? The initial development of the system will be slowed down by fear of its being abused or inadequately safeguarded, resistance coming first from the medical profession and later from the public once they have been alerted to the possible dangers. Although the public already acquiesces in the notification of communicable diseases, or the declaration of disabilities when applying for a driving licence, they will at first resist giving confidential and personal information to the authorities when the health or safety of others is not directly at stake. Patients may try to protect themselves by expressing their more intimate problems in a confidential and unrecorded conversation with their doctor. In all countries, the wealthy classes will tend to ensure that their own medical dossier does not reach the computer, or as little information from it as possible, by using the private health sector. The use of patient data banks is likely to be hotly debated for many years.

In a democratic country, data banks can only develop once the medical profession and the public have been properly informed and reassured about their use. Therefore adequate safeguards must be built into the system, both to ensure that data are not used against the patient's interests and to protect the confidential nature of the doctor-patient relationship. A regulatory code, backed by legal measures, will be carefully worked out to ensure that information is provided from the computer under precise conditions defined so as to protect the interests of the individual, for example to doctors designated by the patient. When data are used for statistical purposes, ways must be developed to ensure that anonymity is preserved. Fears about the system will diminish once concrete guarantees have been established and when its advantages have become widely understood.

Regional information centres will revolutionize the doctor's work by providing a vast amount of information at his fingertips. The computer, far from taking over and impairing his professional freedom, will serve as a highly efficient tool enabling him to diagnose and treat his patients more rapidly and accurately. Often it will detect or suggest previously unsuspected disorders, making health care more effective, but more complex and inevitably more expensive.

Further education of the health professions will be helped by audio-visual teaching methods, including films, video-tapes, and tape cassettes for use in doctors' cars and offices, for which special library facilities will be provided. Closed-circuit television will be installed in all major health facilities for teaching purposes. Radio and television broadcasts for the health professions will reduce the time required for new knowledge to be disseminated; some of these programmes may be made exclusive to their intended audience by means of a key, combination number, or other device on the receiving set. Further training in specialties will be aided by programmed learning courses. Teaching material for these various methods could be prepared by university medical faculties in collaboration with the official bodies of the health professions, who will also control the renewal of licences to practise, this being conditional upon a stipulated amount of further education being received each year. The pharmaceutical industry will continue to provide material and facilities for further training. Advice on the selection of material will be given by governmental agencies and international organizations. Health authorities may try to use educational programmes to influence the practice of medicine, for example by controlling information on new pharmaceutical products, albeit with advice from the medical profession, in attempts to promote drug safety and efficacy and to reduce wastage. Agencies that have to pay the bill for medical treatment, such as health insurance programmes, will help in advising on the choice and dosage of drugs. Programmes will be formulated and run by specialists in medical education, trained in pedagogy and the latest teaching methods and advised by specialists in the relevant fields of health care.

## Health Information and Education of the Public

With increasing emphasis on disease prevention, health education will aim to teach people to be concerned about their health when they are well and not, as is usually the case, only when they become ill. New attitudes are needed to encourage the public to participate actively in preventive health care. The future task of health education, therefore, is not merely to provide information but to cultivate people's sense of responsibility towards their own health and that of the community. In addition to health campaigns on particular issues of the day, for example alcoholism or drug abuse, information will be given on such topics as how to make best use of the health care system, adverse reactions to drugs, and the dangers of self-medication. A computerized system will be developed for sending information to high-risk groups, detected through mass screening programmes or identified in other ways, on the time intervals needed for repeat check-ups and any specific preventive measures that are necessary. Many people, finding it hard to change their attitudes or behaviour, may become confused or hostile when health education makes demands that seem incompatible with their chosen way of life. In order to resolve this conflict and get the message across, a breakthrough is needed in the techniques and psychology of health education.

The greatest impact will be achieved through the popularization of medicine via the mass media, which will be developed in every conceivable way and will spread enormously within the next decade. The mass media have often had a harmful effect on health education, creating false hopes and fears through preferring sensational news about vaccination accidents, heart transplants, or miracle cures to useful and accurate, if less exciting, information. In future, the quality of medical journalism will be improved, and its accuracy and objectivity increased, through the training of health information specialists who will bridge the widening gap between medical science and technology and the public. Few if any of these specialists will be doctors, since the provision of information is a specialized task for which the doctor is not as a rule equipped, whereas it is relatively easy to train journalists in medical problems. Sometimes working as a team, these specialists will keep well informed on health problems through attending periodic courses and seminars, while having the special skill of being able to popularize scientific information in an attractive and palatable manner. Health authorities may attempt to impose censorship of the material used, either through some independent body, such as a university medical faculty or professional organization, or by setting up a government-run medical information agency. While in most countries resisting such intrusion upon their freedom, the mass media and health information specialists will develop a close collaboration with the health professions in order to be accurate and effective.

All the media will be used systematically and on a far greater scale than today. Radio and television will carry specialized and detailed programmes, often at prime viewing times, as well as health items forming part of regular news broadcasts. Animated cartoons carrying a health message will be common on television films and video-tapes; short films dealing with topical health questions will be shown in cinemas; and weekend editions of newspapers will feature lively articles and strip cartoons on health topics. A variety of audio-visual material will be distributed widely to schools, and to health centres and group practices where patients can watch or listen while waiting for a consultation. International travelling exhibitions on health care and health education may be organized. In addition, health information centres will be set up at the district, regional, and national levels within the health services. They will provide individual and group counselling by allied health personnel on such topics as family planning and infant care, and provide reading material, tapes, and video-cassettes for consultation. Educational material for the mass media and the information centres will continue to be provided by governmental agencies concerned, for example, with child health, occupational health and safety, rehabilitation, or food and drugs; by governmental bodies responsible for national health insurance; by official bodies of the health professions; by the universities; by the World Health Organization; and by voluntary organizations such as the Red Cross and national cancer or heart associations. An expanding source of health information will be public discussions and debates on topics of medical importance, especially those with ethical implications, for example computerized information centres, euthanasia, eugenics, and new forms of treatment known to carry certain risks.

Governments will inevitably be involved in health education, with a government-sponsored and financed health education council or similar body responsible for planning and co-ordination on a national level. Non-governmental organizations, encouraged to participate within the frame-work of the overall national plan, will play a valuable role in creating motivation as they cannot be suspected of serving official doctrines. More-over, governments may have a conflict of interest that makes them less effective; for example, if they are receiving substantial revenues from the sale of alcohol and tobacco, they may be reticent in sponsoring campaigns to limit their use.

Health education will develop as a separate discipline and not merely as an adjunct to other health measures. Nevertheless, attempts will be made to incorporate it systematically into medical practice. At the indi-vidual level it will be provided by the general practitioner, through ad-vising his patients on adapting their life-style, or on any special preventive measures needed to protect and promote their health. Trained, up to now, more to receive than to impart information, doctors will abandon their traditionally secretive and authoritarian role once medical school curricula include the teaching of effective communication.

Some health education will be aimed at selected target groups. These may be workers in the same factory or residents of the same village or housing complex, who will be advised about the health aspects of their particular environment. Employers, managers, and trade union leaders must be convinced scientifically of the health and economic reasons for applying certain health measures at work. Other groups include families, and high-risk groups detected by mass screening programmes, who will receive information from their general practitioners. As children form an important target group, parents and teachers will be taught to provide health education from the earliest age. Compulsory and systematic programmes will be incorporated into school curricula, covering such topics as nutrition, dental hygiene, drugs, and sex. Health education divisions of health departments will be responsible for instructing teachers, including a nucleus of specially trained health instructors, so that health education will become as widespread as other aspects of education. Propaganda will be directed to all age groups, as education at school is not enough to ensure life-long, health-promoting behaviour.

# 11 | Costs of Health Care

Health expenditure will increase by leaps and bounds over the next twenty years, as a result of an enormous rise in costs, the widening concept of health, and growing public expectations and demands. As fast as new medical services become available, new needs are perceived. Universal access to health care, automated multiphasic screening programmes, expanded rehabilitation services, and the increasing complexity of hospital treatment will cost huge sums of money, only partly offset by greater efficiency due to automation, the use of allied health personnel, and improved management techniques. This will raise the question of priorities and may involve the temporary rationing of services. Priorities will sometimes be discussed in a way that has not been customary so far; for example, should money spent on prolonging the lives of people over 75 years of age be limited, in favour of more active programmes to reduce accident rates or the number of handicapped children? Should money be spent on artificial kidneys for patients with chronic renal failure, or on multiphasic screening programmes for the seemingly healthy population? Discussion of such problems may become intense and take on political overtones within the next five or ten years.

Systems for financing health care are likely to evolve out of existing ones and therefore to vary from one country to another; from a comprehensive and universal national health service in the United Kingdom, for example, to mixed governmental and private insurance in the USA. In all systems of financing, a greater governmental contribution and the enlargement of social security mechanisms appear to be irreversible trends. Ideological criteria for distributing the burden of health costs will tend to be based on egalitarian concepts, such as the right of each individual to the best care available. Whatever their political structure, countries will attempt to close the gap between two types of health care, one for the rich and one for the poor.

In some countries, the State will cover personal health costs directly. Governments will also tend to assume responsibility for financing prevention, early detection, and surveillance programmes; the monitoring of environmental pollution levels; health facilities and equipment, including computers and automated laboratories; medical information services; and health education. The government's contribution to health costs will be paid for largely out of various forms of taxes. Sophisticated medical technology could become so expensive that no country will be able to afford to use all of the techniques that are developed. Governments may then exert control over whether and when certain extremely expensive techniques are used. However, the distribution of health expenditure must in future be viewed, not only from the national perspective, but in terms of new regions that are being created across national frontiers, and of international communities such as the European Economic Community.

By 1990, the costs of health care in most countries will largely be covered by a tax-supported national health service, or a national health insurance programme that is obligatory for the entire population. Included will be the full costs of serious and prolonged illness, preventive care and surveillance following the early detection of disease or high-risk states through mass screening programmes, doctors' services, prescription drugs, glasses, and other medical appliances. National health insurance will provide extensive cover against accidents and may partly cover the costs of dental care. It will be financed, in the case of the working population, mainly by the beneficiary and his employer through a payroll tax proportional to taxable income, while the aged will have an insurance programme financed during their working lives and the poor will receive free health care.

Two developments in the financing of health insurance will contribute to more satisfactory care for the lower income groups in particular. Firstly, the benefits of the national insurance programme will be made uniform rather than proportional to the size of contribution; and secondly, the system of reimbursement of expenses for private health care will evolve into the entire provision of health care and insurance by the State. Most countries will retain or re-introduce some financial responsibility on the part of the individual, in the form of a small contribution to discourage unnecessary or excessive use of the health services. This contribution may be graded according to income and take the form of a share in the costs of minor health items, cosmetic surgery, and other elective treatment. In some countries, a national health insurance programme will evolve out of a government-subsidized, voluntary insurance scheme, which may include special arrangements for financially deprived groups. Totally private insurance schemes will persist to some extent in many countries, to provide the extra care some patients may want and can afford.

By 1990, the total health budget will rise to a plateau level equal to about 9 % of the Gross National Product. Some three-quarters will be accounted for by health care in hospitals, health centres, and other facilities. Total expenditure on all aspects of health care, including social welfare and other fields affecting health indirectly and not paid for out of the health budget, for example environmental protection, may well rise to between 35 % and 40 % of the Gross National Product. Although the per capita expenditure on health care will increase, largely as a result of generalized health insurance, the overall rise in expenditure will fail to keep pace with even more rapidly mounting economic requirements. There will always be a relative lack of financial resources, producing a lag between what is conceived as desirable and what is achieved in practice.

In most countries, the trend will be towards a relative growth of preventive and rehabilitation services, especially where these are up to now the least developed, and a relative decrease in expenditure on therapy. However, the proportion of the health budget spent on various aspects of intervention is difficult to predict accurately, for a number of reasons. Not only is the distribution of expenditure liable to be influenced by such unpredictable factors as public attitudes, political decisions, and new developments in medical technology, but prevention, detection, treatment, and rehabilitation are to some extent interdependent and separated by unclear boundaries. The early detection of subclinical pathology, for example, may lead to the treatment of asymptomatic conditions with a saving on the treatment of established disease; or the early detection and surveillance of angina pectoris, hypertension, and diabetes may save expenditure on treating heart attacks, strokes, and cataracts. Although the distinction between treatment and rehabilitation is clear in the case of most communicable diseases, it is often blurred in such conditions as chronic rheumatic fever, hemiplegia, and mental illness. Moreover, many aspects of prevention and rehabilitation will fall outside the health budget as the concept of health care widens. The cost of each type of intervention is not always in proportion to its effectiveness or public health importance. Certain forms of treatment, such as organ transplants, will inevitably be expensive, whereas others, for example automated multiphasic screening programmes, will cost relatively little once they have been set up. Controlled trials and cost-benefit analysis are needed to assess the relative values of prevention, early detection, treatment, and rehabilitation in order to establish meaningful priorities.

Soaring health costs will induce governments to further encourage prevention in an attempt to offset rising expenditure on treatment, while general awareness of the importance of prevention will increase enormously. Employers will exert pressure once they realize the economic advantages, for example through reducing absenteeism. A better informed public will also demand services for the prevention of cardiovascular diseases, or for the early detection of cancer or diabetes. Despite a time lag in putting ideas into practice, partly out of the fear of diverting funds from essential therapeutic services, expenditure on preventive care may double between 1970 and 1980, largely as a result of setting up automated multiphasic screening programmes. Governments will invest in health education as a potentially effective means of prevention, aiming to persuade the population to change long-accepted practices, such as smoking and excessive alcohol consumption, or to accept such measures as the fluoridation of drinking water, healthy diets, and the wearing of crash helmets or car seat belts. Expenditure will also increase for controlling drug abuse, occupational diseases and accidents, and road accidents, and for preventing viral and venereal diseases through compulsory vaccination programmes and the development of new vaccines. Other types of preventive health measures will be developed that fall outside the health budget, including environmental protection, town planning, and the development of 'leisure hygiene' through the provision of facilities for sport and outdoor recreation, such as public parks.

Expenditure on therapy, while rising more slowly than that on prevention or rehabilitation, will continue to account for over half of the health budget, largely as a result of the rising costs of hospital care. The amount spent on hospital treatment will be influenced by an increasing number of expensive new techniques, such as organ transplants and vascular surgery of the coronary arteries, although these costs will partly be offset by reducing the length of stay in hospital and by more efficient organization, aided by the greater use of allied health personnel and automation. Treatment expenditure could, however, evolve in an unpredictable manner, since governmental controls may be applied in one country but not in another; for example, the list of authorized drugs may be restricted, or control exercised over the use of expensive surgical techniques. Authoritarian regimes could in this way reduce the amount spent on therapy, whereas such expenditure would continue to increase enormously under a more liberal system. Treatment expenditure will tend to increase as new forms of therapy become available, for example for cancer and mental illness, and chemotherapy of viral diseases. Greater expenditure will be incurred for traumatic surgery, owing to an increasing number of road accidents, and for the expanded use of mobile intensive care units in the treatment of cardiac disease, accidents, and poisonings. A major need will persist for therapeutic relief and comfort in those common degenerative diseases that cannot be prevented or cured; this need will grow in importance with the aging of the population. It will in general be easier to obtain funds for new types of treatment that appear spectacular and give quick results, although some forms of prevention, too, such as immunization against viral hepatitis and the venereal diseases, will also produce convincing and rapid results. The rise in treatment expenditure will be slowed down by increased activities in prevention, early detection, and rehabilitation and the lowering of drug costs due to governmental controls over distribution, profit margins, advertising, and prescribing habits.

More will be spent on rehabilitation as a result of increasing needs and the realization, in most countries, that far too little is being spent at present. Economic pressure, especially in highly industrialized countries, will encourage rehabilitation in order to ensure a faster return to productive employment. Costs will be borne by national health insurance programmes and will include a guaranteed income during rehabilitation. The final stages of rehabilitation will often be financed outside the health budget, for example housing and long-term care of the aged and measures for social re-integration of the handicapped.

The geographical distribution of health care expenditure within a country nearly always depends more on demands than on needs. In most countries, district hospitals are usually smaller and more poorly staffed in rural communes than in large towns. The present bias in favour of urban communities is likely to continue over the next decade, as a result of the greater political pressure exerted by urban populations and growing interest in the health problems arising from urbanization. Although health facilities at the regional level at present benefit mainly town dwellers, they will be used increasingly by rural populations, whose demands for health care will grow as a result of health education. Health authorities will encourage this trend through providing a special transportation system as part of the health services. By 1990, levels of health care in rural and urban areas will have become almost equal.

The distribution of expenditure on different types of disease varies enormously from one country to another, according to demographic and political factors and morbidity patterns. The rise in expenditure on therapy will be accounted for largely by cardiovascular and mental diseases, cancer, and the chronic degenerative diseases. The aging of the population will lead to increased expenditure in particular on hospitalization, rehabilitation, and treatment of the chronic degenerative diseases. Some people question the assumption that needs for health care increase as a result of an aging population, pointing out that a high proportion of old people may, on the contrary, indicate a high level of health in the community. Nevertheless, the fact that health care expenditure on the aged is at present low, relative to their needs, suggests that it will increase considerably over the coming decades.

# 12 | The Role of Industry

The greatest problem facing the pharmaceutical industry is how to pay for a thorough and effective research programme in spite of increasing governmental controls over drug safety, efficacy, and prices. Research and the development of new products will continue to be vital and indispensable activities of the pharmaceutical industry, to ensure the constant innovations that are needed in order to provide ever safer and more effective drugs. Since universities and research institutes do not as a rule have the financial resources, skills, and technology required for developing a new chemical compound into a clinically usable pharmaceutical agent, the pharmaceutical industry will continue to be responsible for virtually all applied research, from the time a new therapeutic principle has been established up to the development of a new marketable product. Preclinical and clinical evaluation are becoming more complex, with increasing emphasis on drug metabolism and drug interaction. Pharmaceutical research, already highly expensive in terms of cost-versus-benefits, is becoming even more expensive as the simpler problems are dealt with and the more difficult ones remain to be solved. For example, effective agents have been developed against the communicable diseases, but not yet against degenerative, mental, and genetic disorders. As the development of a single new product usually takes between five and ten years and may cost some ten million dollars, it is hardly surprising that fewer new products are being introduced each year. In addition to these problems, the pharmaceutical industry is assailed by ever-greater demands from the government, the public, and the medical profession for safer and more effective drugs, as well as by pressure from the government and health insurance bodies to lower, or at least to stabilize, drug prices. In seeking a solution, the industry will continue to expand its markets into international communities such as the European Economic Community, as well as on a wider international scale, and to increase the size of companies through mergers leading to greater productivity and efficiency.

Despite the rapidly mounting costs of research for smaller economic returns, the funds available for research are diminishing, owing to the control of drug prices and profit margins. Since research is essential for progress, pharmaceutical companies will endeavour to reach a threshold size enabling them to devote sufficient funds for this purpose and hence to ensure their survival. It is doubtful, however, whether even the largest national companies, at least in Europe, will be able to compete success-fully with large international firms, which are far better placed for finding markets, carrying out complex and costly research, and selling their pro-ducts at relatively low prices. The trend will therefore continue towards the formation of larger, supranational or multinational companies. Be-cause of their specialized nature, these firms will tend to diversify relative-ly little, mainly into certain chemicals, dietetic products, and cosmetics, whose manufacture is closely related to that of pharmaceutical products. Subsidiary companies may be set up for the manufacture of these other types of product. Certain governments will nevertheless encourage purely national pharmaceutical companies, because they will be better able to control these firms and to negotiate, for example, over drug prices than in the case of international companies.

Even the formation of giant international enterprises is unlikely to provide a total solution to the problem of making adequate research funds available. It seems inevitable, therefore, that governments will be involved in research, probably in one of four ways. Firstly, they could allow for the costs of research when fixing drug prices; that is, the research that was carried out not only on the particular product being sold, but also on the many other products that were studied at the same time but never reached the point of being marketed. Since, at least in Europe, about 60 % of pharmaceutical products are paid for by the State, either directly or through the social security system, this would increase governmental ex-penditure. A second method is for governments to maintain low drug prices and to subsidize research directly, in the same way as other private industries are being subsidized today, for example the aerospace industry. Many practical problems would need to be worked out for subsidizing international companies, but should not be insuperable. By the turn of the century, it seems improbable that even the largest companies will be able to carry out an adequate research programme without State assistance. Thirdly, governments may orient research through providing subsidies for particular areas of investigation, such as those that have tended to be neglected by the pharmaceutical industry because of their relatively low economic returns. Finally, some agency for research co-ordination could be set up at the national level; fed by obligatory contributions from all pharmaceutical companies, it would distribute funds for research to individual firms according to merit. This system would differentiate, for example, between companies that undertake fundamental research of benefit to the entire industry and those that tend to exploit the discoveries of others. Encouragement could also be given in this way to small firms which, unable to carry out an extensive research programme, limit themselves to substances requiring delicate and specialized techniques, such as certain proteins and hormones of human origin. In addition to these various types of State assistance, the pharmaceutical industry may work out some system of its own for economizing on research efforts and expenditure, for example by dividing research into areas of investigation and allocating these to different companies.

Basic pharmacological research will continue to be carried out mainly by universities and research institutes, rather than by the pharmaceutical industry. Although governments will provide grants and subsidies for basic research, they will tend to cut down such expenditure in favour of allocating funds for health care and improving the health infrastructure. The limited funds available may be directed preferentially to problem areas that could have practical application in health care. Funds for basic research will also come from the pharmaceutical industry, for example through research contracts with universities, and from private foundations. Some private institutes will, like the Institut Pasteur, be partly financed from the sale of their own pharmaceutical products.

Controls over the marketing of new pharmaceutical products are tending to become stricter, covering safety, efficacy, and an assessment of the innovative value of a new drug. These controls may come to include the monitored controlled release of new products and improved surveillance after marketing, particularly with regard to possible adverse reactions. The pre-marketing clearance by drug licensing boards is likely to be made more efficient, however, with some reduction in the time required for approval. Today, governments are responsible for authorizing the marketing of new drugs within their own country, even though there are many products that are sold in different countries, often under different brand names, which are manufactured by a single company. Controls are enforced in each country without taking account, apparently, of those being applied elsewhere. These national measures may evolve into multinational controls, for example within the European Economic Community, or international controls on a wider scale under the auspices of the World Health Organization. At the national level, agreements will be made within the pharmaceutical industry to limit the number of different brands of each drug. Favouring this trend, essential drugs may be prescribed and sold only under their approved names, trade names being limited to certain non-essential products. Promotional efforts will, as a result, be oriented towards emphasizing quality control and will be directed mainly towards those responsible for managing drug distribution centres.

Governments are unlikely to exercise much control over the packaging of drugs, which probably has little effect on prices or expenditure. In the Netherlands, for example, where drugs are sold loose, this does not seem to have led to economies or avoided wastage. The pharmaceutical industry will tend to follow the habit of other commercial enterprises in presenting their products in an attractive manner. The supplying of medicaments through government-controlled drug distribution centres, rather than by the traditional pharmacist, may contribute to a lowering of prices. Whereas certain, relatively harmless products will be sold through automatic vending machines, some of the more potent agents may, in contrast, be restricted to specialist use and no longer be available to all doctors.

Since governments are exerting increasing control over the technical and financial aspects of drug production, one may wonder whether they will become directly involved in production through either nationalizing or competing with the pharmaceutical industry. In Sweden, the government has already taken over a number of companies in the hope of reducing costs, but this has met with little success so far. In future, some moves to nationalize the industry can be expected, but are likely to be discouraged by the growing size and international nature of pharmaceutical companies. Governments will rarely be able to compete successfully with private industry. State manufacturing companies may, however, take over the monopoly for certain products. In Australia, for example, the Commonwealth Serum Laboratories, a wholly government-owned enterprise, is the sole national supplier of certain vaccines and hormones.

The medical equipment industry is still at an early stage of development in comparison with the pharmaceutical industry, but is expanding even more rapidly under the stimulus of rising demands and advances in technology. The use of medical equipment is growing in the areas of diagnosis, especially for carrying out functional tests, and of treatment, using a wide range of prostheses that includes artificial limbs, hearts, and kidneys. Artificial livers and sense organs will eventually be available. Electronic devices will be used increasingly for patient monitoring and for the transmission of ECG's and other data from the patient's home or the mobile unit to the hospital or health centre. Perhaps the most rapid development will be in equipment for carrying out manoeuvers that are at present beyond the scope of human dexterity, using miniaturized, electronic equipment and remote control techniques, for example intra-corporeal television.

The cost and complexity of equipment ranges from disposable plastic syringes to automated laboratory equipment for multiphasic screening. As in the case of the pharmaceutical industry, high research and development costs will lead to mergers and the formation of international companies, although certain, less costly items will be produced by subsidiaries of the drug industry. Governments will follow the trend in drug control, in enforcing measures to ensure quality, efficacy, and reasonable prices.

Certain medical appliances for personal use, such as hearing aids and cardiac pacemakers, will be paid for by the patient, who will be reimbursed fully or in part by the health insurance scheme. Although portable artificial kidneys will be available by the late 1970's, it will be some ten years later before they come into home use on a wide scale. These and other large and expensive types of equipment, such as respirators, will remain the property of the hospital or the manufacturing company and be hired to the patient, who will be reimbursed as for smaller items. Governments will lay down guidelines for the costs of hiring equipment, while some types of equipment may be lent by hospitals free of charge as a national insurance benefit.

During the next twenty years, governments may exercise ever-stricter control over the pharmaceutical and medical equipment industries. Alternatively, industry and government could enter into a constructive and willing partnership, serving the common goal of helping to ensure the highest possible level of health care.

# Conclusions

The foregoing study is based on the use of well-informed opinions in predicting future changes. One weakness of the method, which was drawn to the attention of the collaborating experts, is that it is easy to confuse what is probable with what is desirable. Another problem is that many factors are unpredictable and hence extrapolation from past and present trends can be misleading. The future of health care will be influenced in particular by unforeseen social, political, scientific, and technological developments. 'Opinion technology' cannot therefore be expected to give a wholly accurate and reliable view of the future. Nevertheless, it is certainly a valid tool for indicating probable future trends.

What are the principal conclusions to emerge from the study? Far-reaching changes are envisaged in health care, which is seen evolving in a progressive and rational way rather than undergoing sudden or dramatic upheavals. In parallel with the changing concept of health, the emphasis will shift towards preventive and community medicine and environmental hygiene, in the broadest sense, although no radical solution is foreseen to the growing health problems arising from urbanization and industrial pollution. With the neuroses continuing to increase at an alarming rate, mental health services will be greatly expanded, largely through group therapy and care at the community level. Tomorrow's health services will be based on teamwork and the growth of the allied health professions, the expanding use of automation, and more efficient health planning. In most countries, the trend will continue towards the socialization of health care; it is unfortunate that so few experts from the socialist countries of Eastern Europe participated in the study, particularly as those countries already put major emphasis on the preventive aspects of health care. Whatever the system of care, measures can be implemented only if adequate resources are available. With soaring health costs, the search for ways of establishing rational priorities is coming to assume vital importance.

The developed world can now afford to extend its health objectives to include not merely the control of disease and infirmity but also the attainment of mental and social well-being. What, however, is the concept of health as perceived in the developing countries? How do they view their problems and health services in twenty years' time? One would expect quite different answers to these questions from regions that are not only afflicted by, for example, over-population, vector-borne and parasitic diseases, and malnutrition, but which have far less resources with which to achieve their aspirations. In order to place the present study in its global perspective, it might therefore be of interest to carry out a similar inquiry in a number of developing countries.

Many questions are raised which, in the developed world, are likely to become vital issues during the next twenty years. For example, what changes are needed in the training curriculum of doctors? How can systems analysis and cost-benefit analysis be used to achieve more rational and efficient health planning? What is the value of mass screening programmes, in terms of cost-versus-benefits and their efficacy in detecting specific diseases? How can the health services play an effective role in promoting a healthy physical and social environment? What use should be made of automation in screening programmes, diagnostic procedures, and medical information systems? Can international co-operation be achieved in the licensing requirements for new drugs?

The author has tried to place these and numerous other issues in their true perspective within the overall picture of health in 1980–1990. While the examination of such problems in depth is beyond the scope of the present study, such investigations and the finding of valid solutions appear to be urgently required. But that is not enough. The outcome will ultimately depend on what policies are adopted and how priorities are established. Health is inseparably bound up with virtually every field of human endeavour, from science and technology to politics, philosophy, and law. Its development over the next twenty, fifty, or a hundred years will depend on the evolution of ideas about the nature of human society.

# List of Collaborating Experts

*Aujaleu, Eugène*  Professeur agrégé, Val de Grâce Hospital, and honorary Director-General, Institut national de la Santé et de la Recherche médicale, Paris, France

*Baeckman, Guy*  Lecturer in Social Policy, University of Helsinki, Finland

*Baumgarten, Kurt*  Senior physician and Professor, Second Department of Obstetrics and Gynaecology, University of Vienna, Austria

*Beraud, Claude*  Professor of Hepatology and Gastroenterology, University of Bordeaux II, France

*Berger, Renato* †  Civil engineer; Chief, sanitary engineering services, Ministry of Health, and Chief, maintenance services, Portuguese Institute of Oncology, Lisbon, Portugal

*Bishop, Frank Ivor*  Clinical psychiatrist, Royal Children's Hospital, Melbourne, Australia

*Bonnevie, Poul*  Professor of Public Health and Social Medicine, University of Copenhagen, Denmark

*Breitfellner, Gerhard*  Pathologist, University of Vienna, Austria

*Bridgman, Robert F.*  Inspector-General of Social Affairs, Paris, France

*Brooks, Robert*  Director, National Federation of Austrian Social Insurance Institutions, Vienna, Austria

*Debray, Jean-Robert*  Physician and Membre de l'Institut, Paris, France

*Delachaux, Armand*  Professor and Director, Institute of Social and Preventive Medicine, Lausanne, Switzerland

*Domanska, Irena*  Vice-President, Polish Red Cross, Warsaw, Poland

*Duhl, Leonard J.*  Professor of Urban Social Policy and Public Health, University of California, Berkeley, Calif., USA

*Eldredge, H. Wentworth*  Professor of Sociology, Dartmouth College, Hanover, N.H., USA

*Escoffier-Lambiotte, Claudine*  Physician and Journalist, Medical Editor, 'Le Monde', Paris, France

*Farber, Joseph*  Gastroenterologist, Brussels, Belgium

*Field, Mark G.*  Professor of Sociology, Boston University, Boston, Mass., USA

*Fry, John*  General practitioner, Beckenham, Kent, England

*Gibbs, Wylie Talbot*  Executive Director, Australian Pharmaceutical Manufacturers Association, Sydney, Australia

*Gilliand, Pierre* Social scientist and Director, Office of Statistics, Canton of Vaud, Lausanne, Switzerland

*Gingras, Gustave* Professor of Physical Medicine and Rehabilitation, University of Montreal, and Executive Director, Rehabilitation Institute of Montreal, Canada

*Hazemann, Robert Henri* Honorary Inspector-General of Public Health and Population, Paris, France

*Heller, Geoffrey V.* Medical economist, Consultant to the Chancellor, University of California, and Executive Director, Health Care Federation, San Francisco, Calif., USA

*Holmdahl, Martin H.* Professor of Anaesthesiology and Vice-President, University of Uppsala, Sweden

*Holzner, J. Heinrich* Professor of Pathology, University of Vienna, Austria

*Houssa, Pierre* Chief, Traumatology and Rehabilitation Centre, Brugmann Hospital, Brussels, Belgium

*Hudolin, Vladimir* Professor and Head, Department of Neurology and Psychiatry, Mladen Stojanovic Hospital, and Director, Institute for the Study and Control of Alcoholism and Addiction, Zagreb, Yugoslavia

*Hutner, Rachela* Director, Central Institute for the Further Training of Middle-level Medical Workers, Warsaw, Poland

*Ilea, Teodor* † Director, Institute of Hygiene and Public Health, Bucharest, Romania

*Illiovici, Jean* Director, Division of Social Affairs, United Nations, Geneva, Switzerland

*Jamet, Charles* Pharmacist, Director of Training and Methods, Laboratoires Sandoz, Rueil-Malmaison, France

*Jungk, Robert* Professor of Research on the Future, Technical University of West Berlin, Federal Republic of Germany

*Kleinsorge, Hellmuth* Director of Medical Research, Knoll Ltd, Ludwigshafen, and Professor of Internal Medicine, University of Heidelberg, Federal Republic of Germany

*Lambert-Lamond, Georges* Former Secretary-General, United Nations Research Institute for Social Development, Geneva, Switzerland

*Laugier, Alain* Professeur agrégé, Faculty of Medicine, Saint Antoine Hospital, and Secretary-General, Société de Démographie et d'Economie médicale, Paris, France

*Lee, Russel van Arsdale* Clinical Professor Emeritus of Medicine, Stanford University, and Consultant, Palo Alto Medical Clinic, Palo Alto, Calif., USA

*Lucisano, Bruno* Scientific Editor, 'Corriere della Sera', Milan, Italy

*Milliez, Paul* Professor and former Dean, Faculty of Medicine, University of Paris, France

*Novitch, Mark* Deputy Associate Director for Medical Affairs, Bureau of Drugs, Food and Drug Administration, Washington, D.C., USA

*Oeri, Hans Rudolf* Chief, Personnel Department, Cantonal Hospital, Basle, Switzerland

*Pequignot, Henri* Professor of Internal Medicine, University of Paris, France

*Perret, Claude* Professor of Physiopathology and Chief, Intensive Care Unit, Department of Medicine, University of Lausanne, Switzerland

*Rentchnick, Pierre* Specialist in internal medicine, Privat-docent, Geneva University Medical School, and Editor-in-Chief, 'Médecine et Hygiène', Geneva, Switzerland

*Rice, Dorothy P.* Deputy Assistant Commissioner for Research and Statistics, Social Security Administration, Department of Health, Education, and Welfare, Washington, D.C., USA

*Rusk, Howard A.* Professor and Chairman, Department of Rehabilitation Medicine, New York University Medical Center, New York, USA

*Schipperges, Heinrich* Professor, Institute for the History of Medicine, University of Heidelberg, Federal Republic of Germany

*de Schouwer, Pierre* Director-General, Health Facilities Administration, Ministry of Public Health and Family Welfare, Brussels, Belgium

*Segovia de Arana, José M.* Professor of Medicine, University of Madrid, and Director, Puerta de Hierro Clinic, Madrid, Spain

*Senault, Raoul* Professor of Hygiene and Social Medicine and Director-General, Centre for Preventive Medicine, Nancy, France (participated in the symposium only)

*Serigo, Adolfo* Director, National School of Hospital Management and Administration, and former Secretary, Central Committee for Hospital Co-ordination, Madrid, Spain

*Speciani, Luigi Oreste* Professor of Social Medicine, University of Milan, Italy

*Stockhausen, Joseph* Specialist in internal medicine and social medicine, Cologne, and honorary Professor, University of Marburg, Federal Republic of Germany

*Sundling, Sven* Director, AB Astra, Södertälje, Sweden

*Tschopp, Peter* Professor of Economics, University of Geneva, Switzerland

*Tuchman, Emil* Physician, Vienna, Austria

*Vuilleumier, Pierre* Physician, Lausanne, Switzerland

*Wakamatsu, Eiichi* Executive Director, Medical Care Facilities Finance Corporation, Tokyo, Japan

*Waris, Heikki* Former Professor of Social Science, University of Helsinki, Finland

*Werkö, Lars* Professor of Medicine, University of Gothenburg, Sweden

*de Wever, André* Director-General, Ministry of Public Health and Family Welfare, Brussels, Belgium

*Woodruff, Philip Scott* Director-General of Public Health, South Australia

*Zocca, Augusto* Member of the Executive Committee, Sandoz Ltd, Basle, Switzerland

# Acknowledgements

The author is greatly indebted to Mr Elmer Bendiner for his valuable comments, suggestions, and encouragement during the preparation of this book; to Professor Milton I. Roemer and Mr Sev S. Fluss for critically reviewing the manuscript, thereby enabling him to avoid many pitfalls and to achieve greater clarity and consistency; and to Miss Bethany Naseck for helping to improve the style of presentation, but above all for her unstinting moral support.

# The Author

Philip Selby was born in Bradford, England, in 1936, and received his medical education at Cambridge University and The Middlesex Hospital, London. He is a former staff member of the World Health Organization, Geneva, and of the Institute of Social and Preventive Medicine, University of Geneva. Since writing this book, he has become actively involved in the newly created Sandoz Institute for Health and Socio-Economic Studies.